Jasper County Public Library System

Overdue notices are a courtesy of
the library system.
Failure to receive an overdue notice
does not absolve the borrower of the
obligation to return materials on time.

March '09

Izzy & Lenore

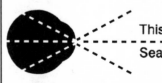

This Large Print Book carries the
Seal of Approval of N.A.V.H.

IZZY & LENORE

TWO DOGS, AN UNEXPECTED JOURNEY, AND ME

JON KATZ

THORNDIKE PRESS
A part of Gale, Cengage Learning

GALE
CENGAGE Learning

Detroit • New York • San Francisco • New Haven, Conn • Waterville, Maine • London

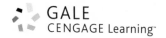

Thorndike Press® Large Print Nonfiction.

The text of this Large Print edition is unabridged.

Other aspects of the book may vary from the original edition.

Set in 16 pt. Plantin.

Printed on permanent paper.

LIBRARY OF CONGRESS CATALOGING-IN-PUBLICATION DATA

Katz, Jon.
  Izzy & Lenore : two dogs, an unexpected journey, and me / by Jon Katz. — Large print ed.
    p. cm.
  ISBN-13: 978-1-4104-0873-0 (hardcover : alk. paper)
  ISBN-10: 1-4104-0873-6 (hardcover : alk. paper)
  1. Dogs — New York (State) — Anecdotes. 2. Dogs — Social aspects — New York (State) — Anecdotes. 3. Dogs — Therapeutic use — New York (State) — Anecdotes. 4. Human-animal relationships — New York (State) — Anecdotes. 5. Katz, Jon. 6. Hospice care — New York (State) — Anecdotes. I. Title.
  SF426.2.K3827 2008b
  636.737'40929—dc22

                                                        2008037800

Published in 2008 by arrangement with Villard Books, a division of Random House, Inc.

Printed in the United States of America
1 2 3 4 5 6 7 12 11 10 09 08

To the staff and volunteers of Washington County Hospice and Palliative Care, and especially to the patients I visited with my border collie, Izzy. I'm grateful to them and to their families for allowing us to share one of life's most intimate moments. Time and again, we met people driven to the very edge of life, often alone, sometimes weary and afraid, and we saw the greatest love, faith, and courage I've ever witnessed.

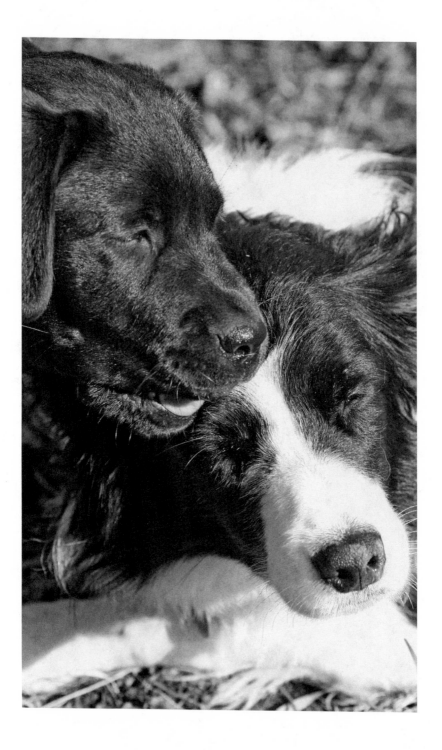

Note to Professor Chernowitz,
and other readers:
No dogs die in this book.

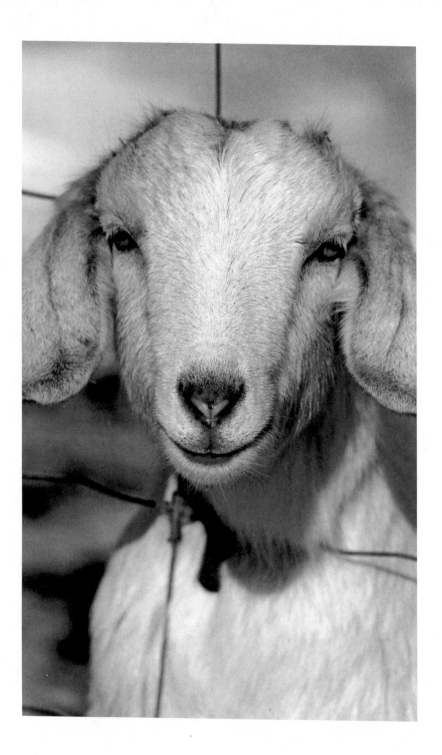

INTRODUCTION

The arrival of three goats — a phrase that, for most of my life, it would have shocked me to write — has altered my morning routine.

Usually my day begins with the sound of donkeys braying joyously, and a bit imperiously, the moment I open the back door. I always have donkey cookies tucked in my jacket pocket — and Lulu, Fanny, Jeanette, and Jesus love their cookies.

But now I have goats, who are even more vocal, and even closer to the back door. Most evenings, before I go to sleep, I have a bowl of low-fat microwaved popcorn, and I bring the leftovers with me in the morning for Murray, Ruth, and Honey. My presentation is not sentimental: I toss the contents of the popcorn bag over the fence and the goats make quick work of it. They love popcorn, so they love me.

The animals on my farm are simple creatures. They love food, anything to do with food, and anyone who brings them food. The goats would love the UPS driver if he brought them popcorn, too.

So on a recent morning, I dumped the popcorn, walked over to give the donkeys their cookies, and scattered some dry dog food out in the barn for Winston the rooster and the gals. The chickens love dog kibble. Accordingly, they love me, as much as chickens love anything.

It was a crisp, late-autumn morning, and sunlight was oozing up over the hill and across the Black Creek Valley, rays streaming across the roof of the barn to the pasture behind it.

The sheep were making their way down the hill, a timeless, leisurely procession. My farm helper Annie, a.k.a. the Bedlam Farm Goddess, brings them hay in the morning, or else I do. So the sheep love me, too. As does Elvis, the giant steer, who appreciates carrots and apples and, now and then, a few glazed offerings from Dunkin' Donuts.

And of course there were the dogs, Izzy, Rose, and the new puppy, Lenore, who bounded alongside me. There's almost always one dog or another beside me. I share Bedlam Farm with three great dogs at the moment. Rose is the worker, Izzy is my soul mate, Lenore is sheer affection.

Rose loves me because I take her to herd sheep. Izzy — well, that's a more complicated story.

Lenore, on the other hand, is not complicated: She adores me because I feed her twice a day and I keep my jeans pockets stuffed with liver treats. She has actually hopped into the UPS delivery truck, ready to elope with the driver, because he brings her treats, too.

Still, it all amounts to a great deal of love, and I take it where I can get it. I appreciate how wonderful it is to start the day with all that baahing, mooing, meowing (I left out the two barn cats, also waiting to be fed), braying, and clucking. I am, at that moment, the center of the universe, at least a small, local universe.

I wish all of last year, or most of my life, were as simple and gratifying as morning rounds on Bedlam Farm. I wish that for everyone.

These animals, I have learned, are unique, each with a distinctive personality, habits, and affections. Getting to know them has been one of the delights of my trek to rural upstate New York, where the population of my farm, Bedlam Farm, keeps expanding. I cherish the predictability of these creatures, their sociability, their contented acceptance of life. I wish I possessed even one of those traits. I'm working on it.

This book is about small things, like getting a new dog that changes your outlook. And about big things, like having a dog lead you places you never imagined going.

About a frightening encounter with mental illness, a struggle to control my mind and to understand who I really am — something I was profoundly shocked to realize I didn't know. It's about coming nose-to-nose with old ghosts.

It's beyond sobering to learn, in late middle age, that you've been running from something your whole life and didn't know it, that certain events shaping your adulthood lay buried so deeply that they could become literally dangerous.

I would learn, in this tough year, some things that wiser people have known for a while: what friendship really means. What family really means. What faith means. How to take care of myself.

And this book is about the remarkable interaction between people and animals, about which so much is said and so little understood. On many levels, I learned a lot.

I've always been wary of people who overburden their dogs and other animals, turning their pets into emotional support systems, the focus of attachment dramas, four-legged psychics and mystic healers. So it was especially startling — challenging, too — to be in need of some of those things myself.

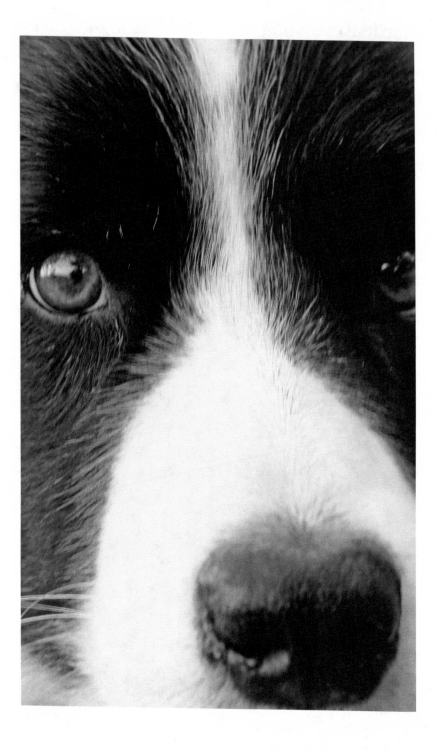

CHAPTER ONE:
IZZY

The place looked like a painting of a farm, not a real one. It lacked the elements of authenticity: rusting tractor parts, rotting hay bales, old tires piled over tarps, the pungent smell of silage.

The farmhouse, astride the tallest of three rolling hills, was in perfect condition, every slate tile on the roof in place, the old clapboards trim and freshly painted. Well-tended flower gardens encircled it.

The fences were all white and upright, the pastures were freshly mown, but there wasn't an animal in sight.

Two large barns on either side of the farmhouse had also been tastefully and expensively restored. The property had the unmistakably crisp look that follows New Yorkers with money.

Nearly a quarter mile from the farmhouse, on the smallest of the three hills, stone steps led up to an enclosure fenced in wire mesh, nearly two acres of ground. Below, at the base of the hill, sat a caretaker's trailer.

Behind the fence, hung with ivy, was a tiny wooden house, almost a miniature farmhouse. This, I thought, must be where Izzy lived, like a princess trapped in a castle tower, waiting to be rescued and brought back into the world.

Flo Myrick and I walked up the hill, opened the gate, and squeezed into the tiny house, perhaps seven feet tall. The windows had no glass or screens, and there was clearly no electricity or heat.

Inside, a worn, smelly, dog-hair-covered sofa sat in the center of the single room; we saw a water bowl, and two other bowls encrusted with dried food, sitting on a threadbare carpet.

"Izzy!" Flo yelled. "Izzy!" No dog.

The story of a beautiful dog running along a fence all day, on an isolated farm deep in the country, had been passed around so often by people I knew that it had become something of a myth. I'd been hearing about this place, and this border collie Izzy, for months.

I doubted the tale could be true. Why would affluent people buy a purebred dog — two of them, in fact — and then abandon them to fend for themselves? Why wouldn't they find another home for them? How could they leave Izzy to race around an enclosure for years? And if they had, then by now the dog had to be half-mad.

Even the story of the kindly caretaker coming by to give the two dogs food and water, bringing them inside during the ugliest storms, seemed lifted from a fairy tale.

So I was anxious to see these dogs I had been hearing about, but I was also apprehensive.

A few nights earlier, Flo had called and begged me to come look at Izzy, to take him home or, if not, to find another home for him. She'd managed to place the other dog, a gentle female named Emma, with a doctor in Vermont. But Izzy was wilder, more energetic, clearly a tougher sell.

I get a lot of calls like that, and unlike so many tenderhearted rescue people, I have no trouble saying no. I don't want a score of messed-up dogs racing around my farm; I don't want to operate a rescue clinic. It would take a toll on me, on my other dogs, and on my farm. Rescuing dogs is worthwhile, but I'm not strong enough to do it over and over again.

"What you heard is true," said Flo. "I see Izzy two or three times a month. He *is* wild and disconnected, but there's something wonderful about him, too, something great-hearted and beautiful. He is really worth saving." Flo thought all animals were worth saving.

Still, curious, I agreed to meet her on Route 22 and follow her out into the countryside to an enchanted but abandoned farm, and to this strangely elaborate doghouse in the middle of nowhere, home to a mythic dog.

Flo, calling for Izzy, was in her late thirties, fit and vibrant, with bright curly blond hair. "There he is," she suddenly said.

We heard the sound of paws thumping on hard ground, and a black-and-white blur appeared, heading like a bullet in our direction.

Hurtling toward us, Izzy ignored me and jumped up on Flo, whom he clearly recognized. I got a quick look at him.

He *was* beautiful — long and graceful, a bit stockier than some border collies, but not wide. He was evidently well bred. He was also alarmingly stirred up, eyes wide, spittle spewing from his mouth, head swiveling. And he was filthy, his coat caked with mud, tangled with burrs, feces encrusted in the hair along his haunches. He looked as if he

18

hadn't been brushed in years; his fur was so thickly matted that I doubted it could be brushed; it would have to be shorn off. His untended nails were curved like talons. Yet he was beside himself with joy to see Flo, rolling into her arms for a brief cuddle before suddenly leaping up and tearing off again to run the fence line, racing two other dogs, also border collies, on the other side. Human connection was no match for the work he did — the running that seemed to possess him. This was not an easy creature.

The others were the caretakers' dogs, Flo said. She pointed to the trench, a nearly two-foot-deep gouge along the inside of the fence that Izzy had dug in his years of running and running.

At night, Izzy and the other border collie, Emma, slept on the sofa in the little outbuilding. He'd seen a vet once when he was a puppy, Flo thought, but not since. As far as she knew, the only human contact Izzy had was with her — she came twice a week or so to bring treats and try to keep an eye on him — and the good-natured caretaker, who fed the dogs and filled their water bowls.

The urbanites who'd acquired this farm initially planned to get some sheep, Flo had heard, so they imported two New Zealand border collies bred from impressive herding lines. The property owners had returned once or twice, locals reported, to check on the elaborate restoration project, which had to have run into the hundreds of thousands of dollars. Then, they barely came back at all. Nobody really knew why; rumor had it they decided they didn't like country life that much after all.

But the dogs remained behind that fence.

For three years (longer for Emma), beautiful, sociable Izzy dug this deepening trench. On the most brutal subzero winter nights, the caretaker brought Izzy and Emma into his own trailer. But since the dogs weren't housebroken, that didn't happen often.

When the absentee owners eventually gave up on the farm and decided to sell it, the caretaker frantically began looking for a home for the dogs, enlisting Flo and her friend Amy, who were active in animal rescue. They started calling me.

I didn't need another dog. I almost never really do. I had my hands full at the time with Rose and two Labs, Clementine and Pearl, who was older and still needed extensive rehab for her surgically repaired legs. Plus, I had the farm and its burgeoning population to attend to.

So I'd put the women off at first, and didn't return their calls.

Then Flo reached me, sounding more insistent and alarmed. Izzy's fate was becoming urgent, she said; the farm was under contract to be sold. The dog behind the fence had to leave his enclosure. I winced at the thought of his going to a shelter, but it was sounding like that's where he'd wind up.

"Jon, I just want you to come take a look at this guy," Flo urged. "I just have a feeling you'd do well together. If I'm wrong, all you have to do is leave. Maybe you can help us place him somewhere else."

I knew how tireless and persuasive Flo and her friend Amy could be. They'd placed dogs, horses, even burros. But this guy — older, wild, unhousebroken — would be a challenge, even for them.

And for his new owner, if they could find him one. She'd brought a number of people to see him, Flo said, but all had turned him down. He was too hyper, too dirty, he'd never lived with people.

Orson, the border collie I'd had to put down a couple of years earlier, was a wonderful dog, bright and beautiful and loving, at least to me. But he had been damaged in ways that I — and a bevy of behaviorists, vets, and trainers — couldn't understand or fundamentally alter. Some dogs never recover from early trauma, or fall victim to breeding and genetic disorders. Others, with the right care and training, can rebound. Which of these scenarios would be true for Izzy was impossible to say.

Maybe these years behind a fence hadn't scarred him so badly. Dogs are highly adaptable, I theorized. Running half the day, getting fed regularly, having a canine companion and some shelter — that might not be so dreadful a life for an obsessive border collie. It was what this dog knew, what he was used to. Dogs can't know what they're supposed to want, or imagine what might otherwise be possible; they live in the moment, accepting the reality around them.

But if he *was* a troubled creature, damaged or barely trainable or aggressive, did I have the time to work with him? The skills? The temperament?

Still, how could it hurt to take a look? I had a farmer friend who often said he might be interested in a border collie, if the dog could work. I would check him out.

As Flo and I talked, Izzy appeared again, moving almost too quickly to follow.

He was a natural force all his own, high-intensity and hyperfocused, without any mitigating distractions — people, real work, training. He came whizzing past, then whizzing past again, wild-eyed and frenzied, like a one-dog merry-go-round. He no longer seemed even to notice Flo, forget about paying any attention to me.

Dog lovers are mysterious in many ways, unfathomable people. I see all sorts of humans unaccountably taking on all sorts of dogs: Sometimes it works, and sometimes it doesn't. There's no dog lover without a heart that's broken at times, and at other times full. Loving dogs invariably means challenges, lucky breaks and good matches, losses and disappointment. That's the drama of it.

Izzy's story seemed a simple one, a classic: Sweet, beautiful dog in need of home finds dog lover recovering from loss of much-loved canine companion. It's only that straightforward in retrospect.

Of course, there was no way I was going to leave this dog to run that fence. I didn't know if I could keep him, though. If I could, it could be extraordinarily worthwhile. If I couldn't, I'd find someone who could.

My heart was thunking. Something important was happening, I could sense it. I wasn't sure this was my dog, but I would spring him anyway.

I pulled a leash from my pocket and told Flo I'd take Izzy home, clean him up and get him checked out by the vet, then try to find him a home.

So Flo waited, then leaned over and grabbed Izzy as he whooshed past, and I got the leash affixed to his collar. Izzy seemed startled and frightened; clearly he'd never been on a leash before. He pulled and jumped and tried to flee. Flo and I wrestled him toward the gate, but he put up a strong fight. Muddy, wet, and foul-smelling, with bits of feces and mud and burrs flying off him, he raked my arms and hands with his long nails.

Izzy wasn't aggressive, but he seemed dangerously panicked, with a wild-animal quality that I'd never really seen before in a purebred dog. He looked almost desperately at Flo, then back at his fence — which I realized at that moment was the boundary of his world, his life, his work. I was dragging him into the unknown.

"Easy, boy," I said, but he had yet to make eye contact. He was frantically struggling to get back to the enclosure, to get free of the leash, to get away from me. I couldn't reassure him, only grab him and, with Flo's help, hoist him into the rear of my Blazer.

I offered him a treat; he didn't even notice. But he lay down in the back of the car and showed me his belly, and I crouched low to get a better look. His teeth seemed fine; his weight was perfect, his muscles firm. But he was a mess behaviorally, more like a feral animal than a domesticated dog.

I probably wouldn't be keeping him for more than a few days. Maybe I should just take him straight to the vet and leave him there until I found him an owner? I knew a border collie rescue group that would come get him, evaluate him, re-home him; I wouldn't have to get involved. I couldn't imagine living with Izzy on the farm.

The ride home was a nightmare. As we pulled away, Flo mentioned that Izzy probably hadn't been in a car in years. She was right: Izzy began vomiting and having diarrhea almost from the moment I stepped on the gas.

Back at Bedlam Farm, he jumped out of my car in the driveway, took one look at the donkeys, pulled free from his collar, and bolted off down the dirt road. It took two hours and heroic maneuvering by Rose to chase him down, get him back into the car and home.

He was a nightmare, aroused, eager to run, confused and frightened by everything — me, the animals, cars, life. It took months to bring him under control, train him, connect with him.

My friend Maria says there's a sadness about Izzy, and I think she's right. Nowadays he's genial and charming, eager to please, full of affection. Yet his story has its share of melancholy, and at times you can almost see it: a sorrow in his eyes, sometimes a fear of loneliness, a sense of having suffered.

Dogs don't experience the kinds of emotional ups and downs that humans do, so far as we know, and they're not thought to have much sense of time. Yet I suspect it was difficult for so devoted and social a creature to be alone behind that fence day after day, year after year, without human companionship. I wonder if he doesn't recall that time in some canine way, if there aren't echoes and images of it in his head.

In his first months with me, he was a wreck — anxious, instinctive, untamed. Left alone, he was smart and strong enough to tear the house apart, and he did his best.

He dismantled crates, ate a panel off the living room wall, went over, under, and through fences to try to get to me.

He was bright enough to anticipate my moves, and several times as I got into the car, I glanced in the rearview mirror to see a tail behind me, even though I'd just left Izzy safe in the house or fenced yard. Had I not looked, I would surely have run him over.

Two or three times, as I was riding a four-wheeler into the woods, he popped up out of nowhere, suddenly running alongside me, so startling me I nearly steered into a tree.

I took him through basic calming and obedience drills for months, but mostly I felt like a janitor, cleaning up his many messes. Even though he always wanted to come along, for weeks he vomited or had diarrhea in the car. And around the house. And in crates. I took to carrying cleaning supplies wherever we went.

He raided the kitchen counter. He raided the garbage can. He would have pilfered food from the other dogs had not Rose and Pearl set him straight.

It was unsettling, because for years I'd tried almost every conceivable training approach with Orson, whom Izzy resembled so strongly. We'd done calming training, obedience training, positive reinforcement, sheepherding. I'd consulted trainers and behaviorists, regular and holistic vets, even a shaman. Orson had Chinese calming herbs and acupuncture. And some of those methods and techniques had enough impact that I felt we'd turned the corner, only to come upon another corner. I deeply hoped to do better this time.

Slowly, after training, socializing, bonding,

we did do better, Izzy and I. The wild animal was subsumed by the companionable dog beneath. Our connection grew stronger, so that he grew more responsive. He paid more attention to me once he knew and trusted me, and it became much easier to communicate with him, and to train him.

He grew fond of my wife, Paula, who was often back in New Jersey, teaching in New York City and researching her own book, driving up to the farm whenever she could. He came to like my friends.

His real nature emerged, undamaged after all, perhaps even protected by his isolation from well-meaning humans. If nobody much had helped him, nobody had really hurt him either. The newly visible Izzy was, in an odd way, pure, unscarred. He'd been waiting, but he hadn't been mistreated. His good breeding and sound nature were largely unscathed.

He was, it turned out, a fine dog. A sweet dog. A dog highly attuned to people, to their needs, and capable of responding with attention and affection.

I can do things with this dog, I thought, things that don't necessarily involve herding or competition. This was a dog that could accompany you on a mission, if you wanted to undertake one. And I wanted to.

■ ■ ■ ■

If you spend time around breeders, rescuers, trainers, vets, shelter workers, you hear this expression now and then: Someone's hit the jackpot.

It means some matchmaker has scored: A dog and a human have found one another and mesh beautifully, embarking on one of those great interspecies love affairs. A number of elements need to fall into place — a person and dog that need and complement one another, that intersect at the right time and fit snugly into each other's lives.

Sometimes when you wait for something, it arrives and proves worth waiting for.

I think I lived for some years behind my own sort of fence, running and running without getting anywhere much. However this story ends, for either of us, it's already a beautiful thing. Izzy and I lucked out: We hit the jackpot.

I'd had an inkling of this when I first took Izzy to see a vet, my friend Jeff Meyer in Granville, a few miles north of the farm. Izzy was cowering on the floor, glancing at me nervously, still only semidomesticated at that point. But Jeff surprised me: He turned to me and said, "You've got a fine dog there, Jon, a keeper. He's going to be a great dog for you."

This wreck of a canine? "Why do you think so?" I asked, relieved that someone else thought my war with Izzy worth fighting, but startled to hear him say so.

Jeff simply said he'd seen the moment when Izzy turned to me and chose me, decided to be my dog. He saw this happen from time to time, not often, and while he didn't know how or why it occurred, it was unmistakable. I found this an odd statement — Jeff wasn't any sort of mystic — but I decided to believe it.

But if the first time Izzy made a choice was in Jeff's office, the second and more important time came a couple of months later.

We were sitting together in the meadow in early summer, watching Rose work with the sheep, always an impressive sight. Izzy turned expectantly to me, as if I had given him a command, though I hadn't. I was just sitting next to him, stroking the top of his head, which he loved.

I saw him close his eyes. If he were a cat he might have purred. The contact, the place, the moment seemed to bring him such pleasure, as if this were precisely what he'd been waiting for behind his fence all those years. He plopped his head into my lap and simply calmed down. It was almost as if he'd decided he was safe, that he understood life here, grasped the simple rules, and was now willing to abide on the farm in peace.

He stopped having accidents in the house after that (and hasn't had one since), ceased his Houdini-like escape attempts, settled into happy domesticity. He was suddenly perfectly willing to be crated. He never chewed or damaged a single thing that wasn't his. He loved riding in the car. He wanted to go everywhere with me, and did. He slept under my bed.

He simply became my dog.

I walk into the kitchen for a cup of tea; a piece of leftover bread crust sits on the counter. Without looking down, I pick up the crust and hold it down by my thigh. A shadowy, furry form slithers quietly from under the kitchen table, carefully removes the bread from my hand, then vanishes again.

I write a few lines and then reach down into the well of my desk. A dog's soft head is instantly in my hand. I pat him, and go back to work for a bit. A little later, when I move into the living room to read, I soon spot a tail poking out from beneath the chair.

I prepare to drive to my favorite hangout to meet a friend for dinner. Rose recedes into one of her lairs in the house. She's not much interested in leaving the farm; she'd rather sit in the house or yard, keeping an eye on things. But there's nothing Izzy prefers to hanging out with me.

He follows me out the door, and when I say, "Truck up," hops into the backseat. Sometimes he stays there for the ride; usually he soon commandeers the passenger seat, resting his head somewhere near my right hand. He doesn't bark or protest or chew while I'm gone. When I leave the restaurant, sometimes two or three hours later, he's curled calmly on the driver's seat. Then we drive home, and I rarely stop to think that not long ago he couldn't ride in a car at all without throwing up.

He's made friends at Gardenworks down the road, at the Mobil station in town, and at the doctor's office. He's even getting pretty decent at herding sheep, accompanying Rose and me on our morning herding lessons. Sometimes he goes out to work with Rose; sometimes he lies down to observe.

When I send him out alone, he's begun to show off some pretty classy moves; he has a big, beautiful outrun and keeps a good distance. He gets the idea of moving the sheep toward the training pen, or down to the hay feeder. More lenient than the no-nonsense Rose, however, he leaves behind some stragglers, including a couple of older ewes who simply can't be bothered.

On the other hand, Izzy's much tighter with the donkeys. He and Lulu, in particular, have some sort of thing going. Out in the pasture, Lulu drifts over and sniffs at him as he lies quietly watching the sheep. He's content to let her nose him, something no other border collie I've had would sit still for.

On the whole, I'd call him a happy dog, even a goofball sometimes. Yet at times, especially at night when I'm reading, or when we're cruising down a highway, he has a wistful way of sighing, putting his head in my lap, looking at me oddly. He watches me, sometimes for a few seconds, sometimes for half an hour.

Maybe that means nothing. But I think a part of him will always be that dog behind the fence, waiting and watching, wondering what took me so long.

Charles Darwin, no less, wrote something in 1873 that makes me think of Izzy. Darwin observed and described specific behaviors dogs use to express affection, including lowering their heads and whole bodies, extending and wagging their tails, and rubbing up against a human and licking his hands or face. These signals are dogs' language, telling us that they're pleased to see us, that we're different from ordinary people, that they care about us.

We respond, I think, because they seek us out independently of our looks or smells, moods or foibles, external successes or failures. We can be angry at them, and they will return. We can be stupid, and they stick around.

They're telling us, in their way, that they accept us, that we can trust and rely on their affection, if we don't abuse it — and sometimes even if we do.

Hitting the jackpot can be as simple as that, and as intricate and meaningful, too.

So my heart has been opened up again; once more the opportunity arises to love a dog. I have a shadow, a pal and companion, a stealth dog who appears and disappears but remains within a few feet of me. He's always there.

From the first time I heard about Izzy, I remembered the notion, common to myths in many cultures, of the animal who comes to us, in our abandonment and isolation, and takes us someplace we can't go alone.

That was the sense I had when I first came

to know Izzy. We were going places, I just didn't know where.

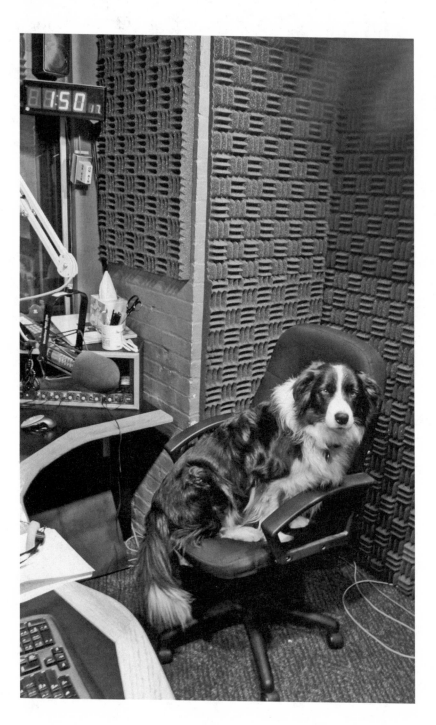

CHAPTER TWO:
GUIDE DOG

The beat-up old Glens Falls taxi pulled up at six. Paula handed me a sandwich and wished us well. I called Izzy; he hopped into the back of the cab. The driver, who usually spent his nights driving drunks home from bars, was unimpressed; if he thought it unusual for a border collie to be taking a cab to Albany, he kept it to himself.

Izzy and I were rushing there to do a live news show for CNN, an interview in the wake of a giant pet-food recall that had dog and cat lovers nearly hysterical, on and off the Internet.

I told the producer I'd be bringing a dog, mostly, I realized later, because I had taken to bringing Izzy everywhere all the time. We pulled up to the Albany studio, were swiftly ushered into a conference room, and would be on the air in minutes.

The other guests, who were in other cities, included a magazine editor who announced that her dogs were just like her children, and a vet talking about how to ensure your pet's food was safe. It was a cable news staple: two or three guests, a couple of minutes of inconsequential sound bites.

The Albany studio had two chairs. I took one, clipped on a mike, saw the red light that meant we were on the air. Only when I looked at the monitor did I notice that Izzy had hopped up onto the chair next to me, and was staring into the camera just as I was.

The host, Paula Zahn, seemed startled, then amused. I answered my question, the other guests answered theirs, and Izzy sat gazing thoughtfully at the camera as if this was something he did every day, rather than something he'd never done. Zahn smiled.

"Should I ask your dog a question?" she said.

"I would," I replied. "He'd probably answer you."

The segment ended, the red light went off, and Izzy jumped lightly down from his chair. We walked out of the studio, through the skyscraper lobby, to our waiting taxi. I rode home with Izzy's head in my lap. Only when we got back to the farm and Paula asked where his leash was did I realize I had forgotten to take one.

This scene has been repeated again and

again, all over the country, as Izzy enters strange spaces as if he's gotten a high-level advance briefing and joins in the activities of the moment. I get lavish praise for my training skills, but I haven't trained him to do most of these things at all.

When I look at Izzy, I often think of the *Where's Waldo?* books that challenge children to find the guy in the striped hat amid a busy throng. Waldo is everywhere, and so is Izzy.

Izzy is, first and foremost, a social creature. Perhaps because of the merciful attention given him by Flo Myrick, the animal-loving blonde who first befriended him, Izzy seeks out blond women and often ends up in their laps.

But then, he's always in somebody's lap, getting scratched, hugged, or cuddled. It's his work, his calling, even more than for my Labs, who are no slouches when it comes to social skills. Izzy is more discriminating and persistent, flashing his brown eyes, sliding his head coyly onto a knee. He doesn't care as much for men, nor is he fond of other dogs besides Rose and Emma, the border collie who shared his long, lonely years.

I've talked before about the Lifetime Dog, who enters your life at a key point and changes it for good. More recently, with the help of my friend Lesley Nase, an animal shaman, I've been exploring the notion of the Guide Dog.

That the term is commonly associated with dogs who assist the blind is apt: My dogs often see things I don't. My early Labs, Julius and Stanley, guided me into a writing life, and then a contemplative one in a cabin in the woods. Orson guided me out of New Jersey. Now Izzy was taking on this role.

He *was* slightly mad when he first arrived. Completely untrained, he didn't know his name, or a single basic obedience command. Having never lived in a house, he tore crates apart, flung himself against doors and windows.

Like other border collies I've known, he saw fences simply as amusing opportunities to show off his athleticism and ingenuity. Most border collies have gone over, under, or through fences in their time. Only the good life keeps mine inside theirs. Why would a border collie leave here? There are sheep in the backyard.

Rose goes months without testing the fence, unless she sees a sheep in the wrong place. Izzy was another story.

Orson had prepared me for challenging times, though, and Izzy's essential good nature made this trouble seem worthwhile. He wanted to be with me, but he'd never been anywhere except the farm where we'd found him, so the world seemed strange to him.

But what the vet had predicted did prove to be true. After a few tough months, things changed. I've rarely needed a leash since. Izzy knows his name perfectly well, comes when called, causes no trouble, rides with me everywhere, is happy within the confines of the farm and the boundaries of my life.

A beautiful, golden-eyed creature, he studied me like a doctoral candidate doing his dissertation on the late-twentieth-century author Jon Katz. He watched what I did, and then joined in; it was as exacting and yet as simple as that. We had no more trouble.

When I go to the barn, Izzy walks alongside and waits for me. When I go into the general store, he lies by the front door. He's not distracted by other dogs (only blond women, it seems), and has never run away since his first day. In fact, we are rarely seen without one another.

I'm not his only beneficiary. He radiates charm and affection, and people see that in him and respond to it. It becomes a circular process: the more he sees people, the more he likes them, and vice versa.

On a recent book tour, we traveled through

the Northeast together. A dog who'd only been in a city once or twice in his life, he matter-of-factly accompanied me to a hotel check-in desk, rode the elevator up to our room, and found a spot beneath a desk or a chair. He wouldn't be seen or heard from again unless it was feeding time, or if I made for the door.

I met a friend at a Chinese restaurant in New York after a TV appearance. Izzy slid under the table, apparently unnoticed, and slept during the meal. When we left, the astonished hosts watched us head for the cash register. We were gone before anybody could say a word.

In downtown Boston, he walked out of our hotel to a tiny patch of grass and eliminated when I said the magic words, "Get busy." Trains, buses, fire trucks, and thousands of tourists and commuters streamed right by, but he didn't seem to notice. He did, however, notice that some green-suited airline attendants from Irish Air, young women familiar with border collies, were staying at our hotel, and was in short order lounging in their laps, getting his belly scratched. By the second day, he spotted their green uniforms in a crowd and made a beeline for them, and the attendants quickly learned his name. Lord, I thought, what a lady-killer.

Along busy Boylston Street, if I was sitting on a bench or taking pictures, he waited and lounged in the sun. He greeted baseball fans streaming toward Fenway Park and tourists getting out of duck boats.

In New Hampshire he befriended vendors at an antiques fair, then waited outside a diner while I ate lunch. Afterward, we headed for the local bookstore, where I was giving a reading. Izzy went in ahead of me, scouting the joint until he spotted the rows of metal folding chairs. I soon heard the usual delighted squeals from the dog lovers, some of whom always came early in the hopes of meeting one of the dogs they'd read about.

Touring with Izzy, I couldn't help noticing the much more restrained greetings that usually awaited me. He always tossed me a sly glance (Who's really the attraction here, pal?) when I caught up.

But so what? However overshadowed, I was delighted to see the joy he triggered, the warmth he elicited, his ability to brighten spirits, as if the lights in the room had suddenly been turned up.

He was a mood elevator. As with a skilled politician, everybody got his due, everyone responded with a smile, and nobody left disappointed. I sometimes felt it didn't really matter what I said at one of these events; as long as Izzy was on hand, I was a hit.

Everybody has his own definition of a good dog; I've had many myself. Rose is a great dog, in that her passion and competence make my cherished new life possible. Orson was a great dog, in that his love and ferocious spirit forced me to change, and to examine myself as a human being.

Izzy is a great dog in a different way: He has an intuitive ability to become a seamless part of my life, a companion in the fullest sense of the term. That he accompanies me through life, when everything about his early years would indicate that he couldn't, is testament to the mystery and adaptability of dogs.

He lacks Rose's ferocious work ethic, or Orson's insane drive and explosive personality. He is different, a calm observer and learner. Perhaps because he waited years for a human to hang around with, he finds his human especially fascinating. Once Izzy has seen me do something — get into a taxi, read at a bookstore — he seems to grasp the nature of the task. So I don't have to watch him; I don't have to call him; I don't even have to think much about him. He is ubiquitous, devoted in the particular way a working dog attaches to a person — completely, and once and for all.

Izzy and I take our act on the road now; he's my advance man.

Last winter, I agreed to speak at a fundraiser for a church in nearby Greenwich, New York. A hundred or so people had crammed into the meeting room: two Girl Scout troops, a number of elderly members of the congregation, assorted animal lovers, a bunch of young kids who'd been promised a chance to pet a doggie.

Our act had evolved; no speaking engagement was fully successful unless a dog was part of it. The speaker himself had become almost incidental. As I hung up my coat, Izzy heard the crowd, walked down the hallway thirty or so feet, went around the corner into the room. I heard the chorus of oohs and aahs as I checked in with the organizers, got a glass of water.

Then, Izzy having warmed up the room, I made my own entrance. He was already casing the refreshment tables, and calculating which of his many admirers would be most likely to slip him a few goodies.

He went from one happy audience member to another, getting his ears and belly scratched, resting his head on knees and on laps. If this had been a bar rather than a church, and he'd worn a thong, people might have stuffed dollar bills inside.

As I was introduced and began my talk, Izzy worked a few more tables. But within a few minutes, he lay down in front of me. Children stepped over him, people brought him food, trays were carried (and dropped). I spoke for half an hour, took questions, and when I finally looked down, he was asleep.

Time to sign books. Izzy lay down under the table; the line of people waiting to hug him was longer than those wanting my inscription.

When we were done, and the goodbyes said, I retrieved my coat, Izzy at my side. "Good-bye, Izzy," the Girl Scouts yelled — until, at a nudge from their troop leader, they said good-bye to me as well.

When I consider his story and how it dovetails with mine, I have to wonder. By what strange turn did this lovely, affectionate dog run a fence for years, until I lost my border collie and could be persuaded to consider another one? What were the odds that the two of us would join forces at that particular point in each of our lives?

Prodded by Izzy's unaccountable appearance in, and impact on, my life, I found myself returning to the idea of myths, mankind's oldest stories.

Before moving upstate part-time in 1997, and then to the farm in 2003, I'd spent most of my life utterly disconnected from the natural world, from the world of animals, and from the power of myth. I was what certain psychiatrists call "existentially lonely," in that, like so many people who live in cities and suburbs, I was cut off from many of the things I now cherish.

I've long been drawn to myths, not only the ancient sagas, but also the modern ones we create for ourselves — Frankenstein, Batman, Spider-Man. I can bore friends and dinner companions by reading aloud from Joseph Campbell, the late scholar and mythologist.

Campbell believed that myths often illuminate our deepest fears, the most disturbed parts of our psyches. Like others, I've struggled with these questions of need, longing, and fear.

The animals in my life, especially the dogs, have shared that experience. Like other symbolic figures in human lives, animals appear spontaneously, Campbell says. They connect with the broken, anguished states of modern humans suffering a variety of disorders of the mind, people disconnected from the communities around them, compulsively fantasizing about the things they lost and yearn for.

We know animals can play important roles in our emotional lives. I've seen the phenomenon again and again, especially in the dog world, with its sometimes obsessive breeders, traumatized rescue workers, overindulgent owners, and compulsive agility and herding competitors. And I've seen it among ordinary pet lovers whose animals fulfill them, providing love, comfort, solace.

In his book *Myths to Live By,* Campbell writes about the point "where myths intersect with animal stories and human lives."

The usual mythic pattern, he writes, is this: Someone begins a quest by breaking away, departing from the local social order. He makes a long, deep retreat inward, backward in time, deep into his own psyche. A chaotic, even terrifying, series of encounters and experiences follows. Presently, if the hero is lucky, he triumphs. His encounters become more fulfilling, giving him new courage. Finally, the hero makes "a return journey of rebirth to life."

Rebirths are nearly a faith for me, and at each turn, each rebirth, there's been an animal to accompany me or show me the way — the Labradors Julius and Stanley, Orson, Rose, now Izzy.

These explorations have often been accompanied by periods of challenge and struggle. They're individual, different for different people, but in mine I glimpse Campbell's universal formula of the mythological hero's saga, which he describes as including separation, initiation, and return.

Thinking of Izzy, of his earlier life, and of our time and adventures together, I kept circling back to the idea of the mythological hero and his mission. That was, without having a name for it, the way I talked myself to sleep every night for years when I was a child.

A hero in myth, Campbell tells us, ventures forth from the everyday world into a region of supernatural wonder, where fabulous forces are encountered and a decisive victory won. I'm not heroic, but I see the hero as simply the traveler, not necessarily a figure of great courage or nobility.

What child would fail to recognize that story? What dog lover hasn't reveled in tales of animals who accompany us through travails and fears?

In her book *Twins*, British psychoanalyst Dorothy Burlingham spoke of the child's desperate search for a partner who will give him all the attention, love, and companionship he desires and provide an escape from solitude. Often this search involves animal fantasies.

An imaginary animal becomes the child's intimate and beloved companion; he is never separated from his animal friend, and in this way he overcomes loneliness.

"The animal offers the child what he is searching for: faithful love and unswerving devotion. There is nothing that this dumb animal cannot understand; speech is quite unnecessary, for understanding comes without words," Burlingham wrote. "These animal fantasies are thus an attempt to substitute for the discarded and unloving family an uncritical but understanding, dumb, and always loving creature."

All this theory seems a lot to put on an animal, even a beautiful and intuitive dog like Izzy, yet it fits almost like a glove. It's how I imagined this dog, even fantasized about him and then experienced him — faithful love, unswerving devotion, understanding without words. I recognize that old and familiar yearning for the uncritical, understanding, always loving companion who will banish loneliness.

So Izzy's sojourn began on his farm, and then he moved to my farm and together we moved beyond Bedlam and out into a wider world. Perhaps I sensed that with him it would grow wider still.

The idea first came from an elderly neighbor I'd met a few times. Her daughter had moved in to help care for her when she developed cancer, and called one afternoon to say that her mother was declining and had but a short time to live. Alice had loved her own dog, a border collie she'd had for years, but she'd had to give him away when she became ill. She still missed him terribly. Her daughter, Della, had seen me around town with Izzy. Would I be willing to bring him over for a brief visit?

I was vaguely uncomfortable about visiting Alice, not sure what to do or say in such a situation. And Izzy, however adaptable, had never really been around sick people. But how do you say no to such a request?

So we drove down the hill one day after lunch, and found Della waiting at the door of her mother's small cottage. Izzy walked in behind me and saw Alice sitting in a living room chair, the tube in her nose attached to a tank of oxygen.

Izzy walked straight toward the older woman, tail wagging, drew next to her, and sat down. He rested his head on the arm of the chair, and Alice reached over to pat him. He held quite still as she smiled and talked to him.

I could see how delighted this woman was, how sincere her appreciation. We spent a half hour with her, and when we left, with Della's profuse thanks, I felt a rush of satisfaction.

We visited several times thereafter. Before long, Alice became bedbound, and less alert, but Izzy capably adapted his routine. He came alongside her bed, climbed up onto it, and burrowed his head beside her outstretched hand. If she was awake, she chatted with him a bit; if not, he lay next to her silently. After ten or fifteen minutes, he hopped off. Della said her mother asked all the time whether this was an "Izzy day."

I'd been looking for something meaningful I could do with my dogs, involving people, not just livestock. But I'd never had a dog with those particular gifts. Maybe I did now.

The funny thing was, I'd been thinking about becoming a hospice volunteer for a couple of years. I'd actually sent for an application, but never mailed it in.

Almost everyone around me thought it a poor idea. I was too busy. It would be too depressing. "You don't need that," said one friend. "It will make it harder to work. It will exhaust you." Even Paula, a hospice believer ever since her mother died in hospice care, worried that I was adding an intense new responsibility, when I already had so many.

Death, I saw, was not something many people want to acknowledge or interact with. I can't say I blamed them. Still, the idea pulled me.

And now I had a dog who seemed comfortable entering a stranger's home and brightening her day. A dog who, unlike me, seemed intuitively to know what to do, how to bring comfort.

Maybe it was time to take the next step. I called Keith Mann, coordinator of volunteers for the Washington County Hospice and Palliative Care program. He delivered the somewhat daunting news: Becoming a volunteer meant hours of training, week after week. Workshops, homework, practice sessions, field trips and visits, evaluations — this wasn't something you merely signed up for. You had to learn a lot, prepare for a lot, be evaluated a hell of a lot.

By now I'd become accustomed to the idea that dogs could influence you, if you were open to it. I was already drawn to hospice work, and I'd been emboldened by Izzy's gift with people, his ability to fit in almost anywhere. A dog like that could do amazing things. With a dog like that, perhaps I could, too. And maybe I should try.

So I made tentative plans with Keith to attend the first class. And by the way, I told him on the phone, I had a dog. A calm, very social dog. An experienced dog. Would hospice be interested in a canine volunteer?

CHAPTER THREE:
IZZY KATZ, VOLUNTEER

The county health department was housed in a small wooden annex in run-down Fort Edward, near the county jail. I parked the Blazer and opened the rear door for Izzy, who disembarked, sniffed around, then paused to look at me, awaiting instructions.

"This way, boy," I said, and he trotted along next to me toward the annex, ignoring a dog being walked nearby, a number of trucks and cars in motion, other people walking through the parking lot.

At the door, he walked inside, scanned the half dozen people in the meeting room, and headed straight for Keith Mann, a muscular, bald man in a polo shirt emblazoned with the Washington County logo. Keith was running the series of hospice volunteer training sessions, held in the annex over several weeks.

Izzy sat down in front of Keith and put his nose in his hand. Keith handed us our name

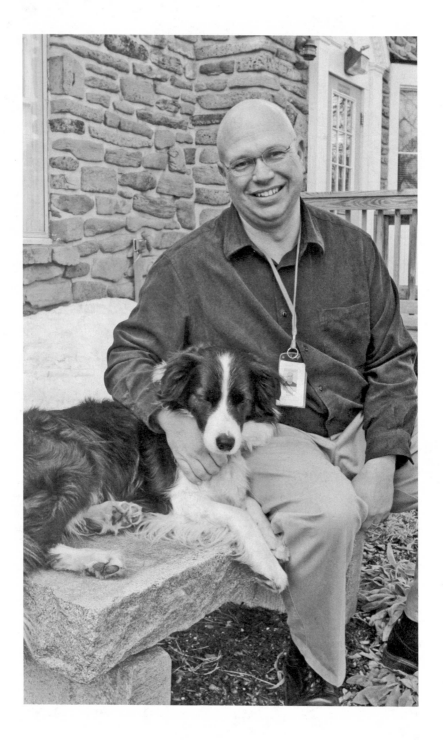

tags, as if it were perfectly ordinary to have trainees with either two legs or four. One said: "Izzy Katz, Volunteer."

This training would test both of us. I had a book coming out, so I was about to start an extended tour. Insanely busy running the farm, I was already harried and drained, struggling to find time to write.

Besides, hospice work was no simple undertaking. The training alone was thorough and demanding, involving considerable role-playing, reading, and memorizing. The volunteer's handbook weighed a good three pounds.

As a former police reporter, I'd seen plenty of bodies, but I'd rarely known anything about the people who died. Here, I would be going into homes and nursing facilities, getting to know people who were failing, getting to know their families, too — and ultimately seeing them die. How would I handle that? Could I do a good job, or would it be one of those projects I sometimes took on obsessively and then, exhausted, had to drop?

I'd gone back and forth about making this commitment. I didn't want to start something I couldn't finish, yet I was learning the hard way how unpredictable and cluttered my life had become.

At first, I'd thought that my busy schedule,

complete with book tour, might cause the program to cut me some slack. Could I really drive three nights a week, for several weeks, to Fort Edward?

But it was clear, as Keith explained the volunteer training to me, that there would be no slack, no shortcuts — and that there shouldn't be. The hospice program needed to make quite sure that the people who entered patients' homes, where the psychological and physical issues were often intense, knew what they were doing and could handle what they encountered.

Accordingly, our training involved talks with social workers, doctors, and other volunteers, field trips to the homes of patients, quizzes — and constant monitoring by hospice staff, alert for weaknesses or problems that might arise. I found my motives questioned again and again. I actually had to defend my desire to enlist.

Keith was a skilled instructor, adhering strictly to his orientation and lesson plans — but he also kept a sharp eye on the volunteers to see how we reacted.

From the outset, at least one volunteer paid rapt attention. Izzy sat staring at Keith throughout nearly the entire session. Sometimes, I did look down to see Izzy dozing. But usually he was locked onto Keith, as if listening intently to every word. I half expected him to take notes.

When we took a break, Izzy followed me outside, where he found a bush to mark, then came back in and approached each of the other volunteers, putting his nose in their laps or on their knees. If they responded, he stayed a while. If they didn't, he moved on. Keith always brought a biscuit or two, so Izzy made sure to visit him during the break.

Several things struck me during our early training. Izzy seemed to have an innate sense of appropriateness. He never disrupted the talks or meetings by barking, whining, or even moving much. He understood that the breaks were a time for socializing but the rest of the session was work.

Six other volunteers were going through the training with us, all arrayed around a conference table, listening to lectures, watching slides, talking about our own lives and our abilities to enter other people's. Through it all, Izzy sat by my side or, often, at Keith's feet, taking it all in.

In a sense, hospice training challenges volunteers to go against the grain of what we ordinarily think of as support, concern, and affection. Normally, if I see people in distress, I try to reassure them, to tell them things will get better, that they're doing fine.

Hospice training teaches you to do the very opposite. In hospice, the ending will always be the same: The patient will not recover; there will be no eleventh-hour happy ending.

Reassurances and conventional wisdoms can't really help the dying or those who love them. Each person, family or friend, will experience death in their own intensely personal way, and I have no tonics for them, no words of cheer. I must leave my own experiences, perceptions, and responses at the door and permit them to face and experience death in whatever way they choose. My role is to listen, and help only in the ways that I'm asked to. It's an extraordinarily sensitive situation.

Yet the work seems so crucial. Hospice workers often talk about the mistreatment of the dying, by which they mean not cruelty but the natural human tendency to shun death, to avoid the dying and retreat from even thoughts or discussions about it.

Hospice families tell me all the time about the pain of having friends stop calling or visiting, of seeing them turn away from them at the supermarket, simply flee in the face of death's awesome finality.

So we leave them, often quite alone, to their fates, to the struggles with our health-care system, to a culture too busy and distracted — or uncomfortable — to pay much attention.

The last thing these people need is some well-meaning volunteer who attempts to cheer them up, offer suggestions on how to die, or tell them how to grieve. All we can do is provide some companionship and comfort along the way. It's a humbling mission.

To bring a dog into these homes seemed an even greater challenge. Patients are often in emotional or physical distress, hooked up to oxygen or IVs, and taking potent medications. Lots of dogs do therapy work, but hospice requires something a dog really can't be trained to do — figure out for himself how to be loving, appropriate, and sensitive to the dying.

To be a hospice dog, Izzy had to be tested by a vet, who issued a certificate attesting to his temperament. I did considerable calming training, praising him for being calm, practicing moving around furniture and other obstacles. We tried him out in several strangers' homes and in a nursing home with a PA system and lots of medical equipment around. And, of course, he attended all our training sessions, where nurses and social workers were watching him carefully.

But the truth was, I had no clear idea how

to prepare Izzy. His own instincts and personality, I thought, would prove more critical than any training in determining whether he could do this work. All I could do was bring him along, into patients' homes and lives, and see what he could offer.

All through the spring and summer, we trekked to Fort Edward, with a sandwich and fruit in a paper bag for me and a few biscuits for Izzy. Keith kept a water bowl in the annex kitchen for him. The volunteers were an extraordinarily generous group of people who seemed quite willing to accept us both, and Izzy was happy to see each of them at every session.

I was daunted at first, by the detailed thoroughness of the training, though I would soon enough be grateful for it. We practiced what to say, what to look for, how to listen. We learned to fill out forms and reports. There was a long list of things to avoid saying — like "Buck up! You'll be okay!" The sessions were wearying, but also gratifying. By the time they concluded, I felt ready.

I can't say I know for certain why I wanted to sign up. Perhaps weathering middle age makes one more aware of death, more thoughtful about it. Perhaps, as my work life intensified, I wanted to make sure I had a grounding, a meaningful commitment to help me see life in perspective, to keep my spiritual self alive. Maybe I wanted see if there was a way to share this work with a dog. Maybe all of the above.

While we were learning, it was hard to avoid the sense that Keith and the social workers were watching us pretty carefully. Whatever our reasons for coming, we volunteers had to talk about them. Stan had just lost his dad. Rita had lost her husband a few years earlier, down South. Donna, it emerged — slowly — had also lost someone, though she hadn't said whom.

On the surface, direct experience with grief would seem a perfect qualification for hospice volunteers, but the staff pointed out that it could also be a problem. We had to set our own losses aside, not add to the sorrow the patients and their loved ones already felt.

Donna and I were paired for role-playing during the second week of training. She was a kindly woman, quietly but deeply religious, and eager to help others. "What better way," she asked, "than to help people leave the world comfortably, with dignity?"

In this exercise, one of us played the volunteer; the other pretended to be a person who had lost someone dear. I drew the volunteer role, which meant my job was to listen, to affirm the feelings I was hearing, not challenge them or add my own or try to change anyone's mind.

Donna, playing the family member, sat opposite me and said she had a sick child, a son dying of leukemia. It was horrible, she said softly, to watch her son suffer, wither, and fade. "I'm not doing enough," she lamented. "I feel like I'm not doing enough, no matter what I do."

It was useful practice, because under normal circumstances I surely would have reassured her, told her that of course she was doing enough, and urged her not to be so tough on herself. This "character" was, after all, sitting by her son's bedside almost around the clock, reading stories to him, administering medications, making him as comfortable as possible. What more could she possibly do?

"How long have you felt this way, that you're not doing enough?" I asked — a neutral question, meant to allow her to communicate but not to talk her out of what she was feeling or dismiss it by suggesting it wasn't really true.

She told me more about her son and his diagnosis, his weakness and decline, about the fact that he might die at any moment while she was right there watching, and how helpless she felt to prevent it.

As she spoke, Donna's eyes welled and her face contorted with grief. I was surprised to see Izzy appear out of nowhere, put his head on her knee, and stare up into her eyes.

Suddenly, I saw what he, perhaps, saw. I understood that Donna was no longer playing a role; she had lived this. She wasn't simply a volunteer portraying a stricken mother. We had moved into the realm of real loss.

I don't know what dogs can see or sense, but I know they can discern things that I can't. Rose sees things invisible to me when she is working with sheep. Izzy had some sort of insight about people.

"I'm sorry, Donna," I said. "How long ago did your son die?"

She put her face in her hands and sobbed. "Five years. Five years." And we were done.

The social workers were pleased; they said I'd handled things well, had been perceptive in seeing that Donna was still actively working through her grief, something important for them — and her — to understand as she ventured into hospice work. And Izzy had been a model of empathic restraint.

We all bonded over those weeks, eating cookies and sharing stories of loss from our own lives. I talked about the deaths I'd seen as a reporter, the two pregnancies we had lost before our daughter, Emma's, birth. I talked, too, about my fear of losing a sense of spirituality in my too-busy life.

We played hospice quiz games and watched hospice movies and talked to a stream of social workers, a warm, funny, intensely dedicated group who reported high rates of burnout and stress among their ranks.

The staff talked a lot about volunteer burnout, too, about the need to prepare for this curious truth: Everybody you are visiting will die, and your job is not to save them but to help them leave with as much comfort and dignity as possible. It will be wrenching, surprising, different every time. It isn't for everybody. There are support groups for us, too, numbers to call, help available.

We were briefed by lawyers and nurses and bereavement counselors. We were taught how to spot trouble — filthy conditions, spilled medicines, rising pain, family members breaking down — and to notify the hospice staff immediately.

We all had fears, doubts, and many questions. Could we bring food or books or other gifts? Pass out our phone numbers? What if we saw family members fighting or patients being mistreated? Could you sense death before it came? What was it like? What were the signs? What if somebody died while we were there? How did people grieve, and for how long? What was helpful and sensitive? What wasn't?

But training convinced me that I wanted to do this. Besides, it seemed no longer purely my decision. Izzy had enrolled. At the end of the summer, we completed our training, passed our background security checks, got fingerprinted (well, one of us). Izzy and I received our certificates and photo IDs at a ceremony complete with cake. We would be notified of our first assignment in a few weeks.

Soon enough, we were on the job. Keith mailed me a hospice assignment sheet, telling me the patient's name and address and condition.

On a muggy, late-summer afternoon, we drove to a small bungalow next to a church on a tree-lined street. I was anxious, going over the training in my mind. This looked like any other house, I thought — then chided myself for such foolishness. Why wouldn't it look ordinary? How easy it was to stigmatize death, to the point of expecting a dying person's house to visibly proclaim its status.

The patient, named Jamie, was eighty-six and in the final stages of Alzheimer's disease.

No longer willing to be touched, terrified of even her own family, she was deemed difficult to handle. The social workers were concerned about her daughter, who'd exhausted herself and her savings caring for her mother. Hospice hoped a dog might help settle her; she'd been a dog lover all her life.

The protocol was rigid. Izzy and I both had to wear our photo IDs, and I had to wash my hands, going in and coming out. We were not permitted to drive patients, to have anything to do with medicines or medical equipment, to perform any kinds of hands-on care. Technically, we weren't even supposed to touch the people we were visiting, although most of us trafficked in illicit hugs.

A former schoolteacher, Jamie had been moved into a first-floor bedroom in her daughter's house. Carol had been caring for her faithfully for several years, but it was growing steadily harder. Jamie slept much of the time, but often yelled or cried out when she was awake. It had become increasingly problematic for the nurses, or even her daughter, to bathe her or change her clothes; she seemed terrified of physical contact and struggled, sometimes to the point of bruising her fragile skin. Carol was worn and weary from the effort. Yet any suggestion of a nursing home was anathema.

Much of the time, the two women were alone in this small frame house, Carol sitting by her mother's bedside, reading or talking to her. Most of the neighbors didn't even know that Jamie was terminally ill, Carol said. They had few visitors. Once her mother had lost her ability to recognize them, friends had drifted away, and family members came by infrequently. She encountered growing problems talking to them anyway, Carol confessed; they seemed to inhabit some other planet.

When Izzy and I came into the house, Keith was waiting for us, as was customary when volunteers paid their first visit to new patients.

Carol, a slight, round-faced woman wearing a lavender sweatsuit, was pleased to see us, welcomed us, and knelt down to pat Izzy. I'd been warned that she was bone-tired and increasingly anxious about her mother, who might sleep all day and then cry out in the middle of the night.

In a tiny, meticulously clean powder room, I washed my hands, carefully and thoroughly, as instructed; Izzy waited outside the bathroom door.

I could see a bedroom at the end of the hall, decorated with family photos and fresh-cut flowers. As we drew closer to the room, I could hear a TV; Carol explained she kept it on most of the time, so her mother could hear voices and feel less lonely.

A beautiful older woman was lying in bed, beneath a summer quilt. Someone had carefully arranged her silvery hair, polished her fingernails, even daubed on a touch of lipstick. She was mouthing barely audible words and moving a bit restlessly.

"This is so great, the dog coming. She loved her dogs so much," whispered Carol as we entered the room.

Carol introduced us loudly and slowly: "This is Izzy," she said. "And Jon. They've come to see you. Izzy is just like Flash. You remember Flash, Mama, don't you?"

Jamie stared at the ceiling and began mumbling. I came to the foot of the bed, looked at Izzy, and gestured to the foot of the bed; he hopped up. "Stay," I whispered, and he sat stock-still.

Jamie seemed unaware of his presence. I waited. Carol was quiet, too. Keith, watching from the doorway, might have been nervous about what would happen with Washington County Hospice's first canine volunteer.

Izzy seemed a bit uncertain, not sure what was happening, looking first at me, then at Jamie. He'd never been in the company before of someone so debilitated, so close to the end; clearly, it was strange to him. Was it smart, I found myself wondering, to bring along this dog, who'd spent most of the first four years of his life alone outdoors? But he looked all right, his ears and tail up, no signs of stress or anxiety. In fact, he seemed to be studying the room, looking carefully at me, at Jamie and Carol, seeking cues.

He cocked his head at me. "It's okay, Iz," I said. "Say hello."

He seemed to get it then, some invisible trigger or instinct kicking in. I hovered nearby, ready to move in quickly if there was trouble. This was a dying woman who didn't want to be touched. Would she be frightened, or perhaps frighten Izzy? How would he respond to a situation he'd never been in, couldn't really be trained in advance to handle?

He lay down and very slowly began inching up the side of the bed. He didn't step on Jamie, or even graze her frail body, just crept slowly alongside her. When he got close to her hand, he burrowed his head beneath it and lay still.

Jamie stopped muttering. Her face looked alarmed at first, then she broke into a slight smile. She didn't look at Izzy, but moved her hand slightly, feeling his forehead and his ears.

"Oh," she said. "Oh." And then, smiling, "Oh, how pretty . . . pretty."

"This is the first time she's said real words in weeks," Carol whispered, astonished.

Izzy kept quite still as Jamie stroked him and talked in disjointed sentences, still smiling. After a while, she drifted off. A few minutes later, her hand still resting on Izzy's head, she awakened and stared at the ceiling, and smiled again. She seemed calmer than when we'd come in.

After fifteen minutes, without instruction, Izzy extricated himself and skipped down from the bed, circling around to Carol, offering her a friendly paw. She kneeled on the floor, weeping, and held Izzy for a long moment. Then our visit was over, the hospice canine volunteer program launched.

"I can't explain how much this means," Carol told me as we left. "For a minute I had my mother back."

We agreed to return the following week. Later, we learned that Jamie allowed Carol to bathe and change her without fear or resistance. Why this would be true was nothing any of us could explain, but something was different.

Outside, Keith shook my hand and leaned

over to praise Izzy. "This works," he said. "This is awesome. Izzy is a natural. You aren't so bad yourself."

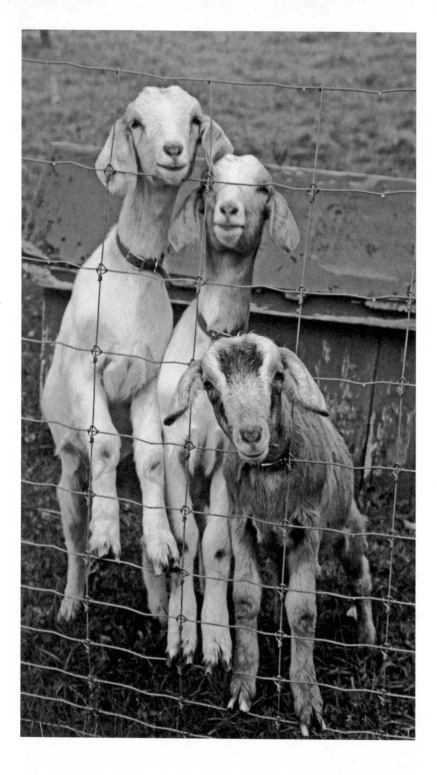

CHAPTER FOUR:
RUTH, MURRAY, AND ELVIS

Maybe Annie was the first one to notice something was wrong. We saw each other frequently — she arrived almost daily in her truck to help with the endless chores of the farm — and had become good friends. But I was also her boss, and she wasn't really sure how to talk to me about it.

We chatted about lots of things, but mostly about our animals — sick sheep, a sore on Elvis's neck, Annie's goats and rabbits.

Every morning we walked the dogs together in the woods and talked about life upstate, the price of hay, and how the farm was faring: Was it time to move another round bale out to the cows? Could we plug the tractor battery into an extension cord so it wouldn't die in the cold? Should Mother the barn cat be permitted into the basement on bitter nights, if we put a litter box there?

I also got to fill Annie in on what I was doing — hospice work, news from Paula and Emma, my growing interest in photography.

At first, Annie and I had been a bit uncomfortable about the way some of our views on animal care clashed. Intensely focused on animals and their well-being, hyperalert to any health problems or signs of unhappiness, Annie was reluctant to put any animal down, ever — even a chicken. Whereas I felt the farm had to be a healthy and working entity, not a rescue haven or veterinary clinic.

Annie always wanted to give grain to the cows and chickens when it was cold, and was constantly urging me to call the vet when something didn't look right. She adopted a parade of sick creatures — rabbits, cats, injured birds — that she found in the woods or along the roadside.

Gradually, we came to an understanding. I gave her a chance to nurse any sick animal back to health; she understood my own philosophy and sense of limits.

As we became closer, learning more about each other's sensitivities and interests, I scoured antiques shops for the farm bric-a-brac she loved — wooden egg holders, root cutters, signs from long-vanished general stores.

She came to understand the issues involved in my work. Sometimes, when I was holed up in my study, absorbed in writing, she would creep in the back door and take the dogs out for a long walk in the woods, and I wouldn't even know she'd been there until the dogs came thundering back in, exhausted and ready to curl up. When I went out on a hospice call, I'd often come back to see a fire already blazing in the stove, the house warm and ready for me to go to work.

So when Annie told me she was worried, it got my attention. "You don't seem to get as much joy out of the farm as you used to," she said, carefully. "You seem very drained."

Paula had been telling me the same thing for a few months. My friend Becky was irked. I'd been neglecting my friends, paying them scant attention, she warned; I seemed distracted, in some other world.

Maybe I was worn down and needed to renew myself. I *had* been feeling depleted — spiritually, intellectually, physically — since the summer's long book tour.

I prescribed for myself daily readings of Thomas Merton, the Trappist monk, contemplative, and author whose books had guided me in the past.

And to rediscover my pleasure in the animals, I decided to do three things right away: I would spend more time with Elvis and let his gentleness soothe me. I might consider a new dog, if I found one that fit well with the current menagerie. And I would get some goats.

Sandy Adams backed her truck into the driveway, a small wooden shelter and two crates piled in the truck bed. My plan had been to put Ruth and Murray, two baby goats, into the big back pasture with the steers and cow, but Sandy noticed the fenced dog run just behind the farmhouse and thought it would be a great spot for young goats: The fence was tight, there was plenty of brush and scrub to eat, and there was the HBO Memorial Lambing Pen.

So Sandy and her husband and kids (the human sort) opened the back of their pickup, cradled the baby goats in their arms, and carried them into the dog run. I could see how fond they were of the two babies they'd raised — though as farmers they of course wouldn't admit that. I could also see they were pleased by the habitat. "Good place for them," nodded Keith. "Lots to eat, good shelter, rocks and trees. They'll be happy here."

The HBO Pen had been constructed during the filming of the movie *A Dog Year,* based on my book of the same name, in and around my farm in 2006. Inevitably, my pregnant ewes were about to give birth the very week the movie crew and its canine cast took over my dairy barn, where I normally kept the lambing pens.

The producers, eager to be helpful, insisted on building me a temporary pen. I tried to tell them that some plywood and wire would be sufficient. It was summer, the weather was fine, so all I needed was a place for ewes and lambs to be kept together for a few days, not the shelter from the elements I would have needed in winter.

No way, said the producers. You need something classy; we insist. So for days, trucks arrived bearing New York–based Teamsters and carpenters ferrying tin roofing, wooden panels, elegant doors.

Within a week, all the ewes had lambed, so Annie and I threw together temporary outdoor pens fashioned from boards and plastic mesh.

But the HBO Memorial Lambing Pen was unstoppable. Construction continued for more than a month — rather, piles of tin and lumber sat in my backyard for nearly a month as the busy Teamsters rushed from one film location to another.

Once in a while, two or three trucks or vans filled with big, muscled, wisecracking guys from Brooklyn and Queens, all cursing, laughing, and carrying mugs of coffee, would pull up. The backyard suddenly rang with hammering and banging, sending the donkeys and sheep scurrying into the pole barn and annoying Rose, who tried to keep tabs on everything that happened hereabouts.

"Yo!" the men would shout to one another. "Lookit the dogs. Hey, donkeys!" As they hammered and sawed, they'd talk loudly about how strange producers were and the odd decisions they made. Then, just as abruptly, a cell phone would ring and everyone would take off, apologizing and promising to return shortly. They didn't, not for days.

Still, the producers were as good as their word, sort of. Six weeks after the last lamb's delivery and two days before shooting wrapped on *A Dog Year,* the Teamsters came by to put the finishing touches on their elaborate project. Then they all shook my hand, gave each of the donkeys a cookie, and climbed back into their trucks, still bitching about producers.

"Nice farm," said Jim, the foreman, before roaring off down the road. "I think I'll stay in Queens, though. No offense." None taken.

Annie and I looked at the strange new structure sitting out back. It was far too big, utterly useless as a lambing pen, yet it didn't have enough space for a donkey or sheep, and a cow would have crushed it in seconds. Could it be used as a doghouse under certain circumstances? I was thinking perhaps it could serve as some sort of storage or garden shed, except that I had four barns, which really provided ample storage.

It occurred to me, a few days later, that while the HBO Memorial Pen might never serve much of a function for sheep, perhaps goats would be a good idea one day.

I'd had goats on the farm a couple of years earlier, two Nubians, but it was one of those matches that just never took. They opened gates, jumped onto car roofs, and whined loudly day and night, annoying the dogs and me.

When one got his horn stump infected, and then nearly died from bee stings, I gave them both to Annie, who had so many goats of her own that I'd taken to calling her the Goat Lady of Cossayuna. Now the two brothers pester her, instead. Unlike me, she loves them for it.

I'd been drawn to the idea of goats because they eat all kinds of scrub and weeds that you don't want around and that other animals won't touch — like nettles, which sting like hell when you touch them.

The problem, I found out, is that goats are as smart as dogs, but pushier and less trainable. They do all sorts of things you don't want them to do, and specialize in going, with great skill, where they aren't permitted or wanted.

Most dogs are dependent creatures, with at least some desire to please humans, if only to procure food, pats, or walks. Goats, like donkeys, are viscerally *in*dependent, with no desire at all to curry human favor, do what they're told, go or stay where they're supposed to. They're irritatingly good at using their noses, hooves, and instincts to make daring escapes.

Though they never seemed to get very far. Usually what ended up happening was that I trotted after the two goats, huffing and puffing, in circles, unable to corral them. Finally I'd fetch Rose, who'd nip somebody in the butt or tail to get them moving in the right direction. If that failed, I just shook a cup of grain or corn and they'd follow me back into the fenced pasture — for a while.

Cut the weeds along a fence, and the goats would spot even small fissures beneath it and crawl out, even if they had lots of grass where they already were and none where they were going. Then, annoyed and anxious, they complained loudly until someone arrived, bearing goodies to lead them back in.

"Why," I always asked the Nubians, "do you want to get out in the first place?" I imagined them saying, "Because we can."

Still, goats have lots of personality. They're playful and social and like to talk to people. Plus, there are all those weeds around the dairy barn that are tough to get to. Goats could, in theory, be useful — and add to the character of a place. And what else was I going to do with the HBO Memorial Lambing Pen?

Having reached this decision, I did what anybody upstate does when he wants something. You tell Cindy at Stewart's, say something at the Bedlam Corners General Store, or stop in at Gardenworks and mention to Meg or Arlene that you might be interested in a couple of goats. Then you wait for the phone to ring.

Mine did a couple of days later. Sandy Adams, Arlene's daughter, lived on a farm in the nearby hamlet of Shushan and bred goats, a Boer/Saanen cross. I knew a little about this crossbreed: they were smaller than Nubians, and calmer. Sandy said her two children raised the goats, showed them at 4-H fairs, spent time with them. These kids (the goat sort) shouldn't be as incorrigible as the others I'd had.

The next day, I drove out to Shushan with my friend Maria. The Adams farm, set on a hillside, was lush and green. The whole family was there to greet us and show us the goat pen, a small enclosure with two or three adults and three babies. The other young goats had all been sold, and if these three weren't soon, Sandy said, they were going to market.

Sandy and Keith were picture-postcard upstate farmers — fit, tanned, courteous. They enjoyed keeping goats. Every summer evening, they let them out for a romp in the yard. The junior Adamses had been caring for goats for years in exchange for allowances, just the sort of thing suburban kids were rarely able, or asked, to do.

But Sandy was also decidedly unsentimental. There was little doubt that the goats would be going to a livestock auction if someone didn't buy them.

She let the goats out, and they pranced around a bit, then hurried back into the pen to be with their mothers. The adults were smallish, perhaps three feet high, alert and inquisitive but relatively calm. I let Izzy out of the car and he took one look up the hill at the dancing goats and ran under the car, peering out fretfully.

Sandy had named one of the babies Honey; the others were as yet unchristened. They were good goats as goats go, she assured me, responsive, curious but not too curious, peaceable. They didn't need much room — hers all slept bunched up in a hut the size of a small doghouse — and loved nettles and scrub and weeds, along with grass and hay.

I told Sandy I'd take the two unnamed goats, though they weren't unnamed for long. Paula proposed calling them Ruth and Murray, after her mother, who'd died a few years earlier, and her father, Murray, alive and well in Vineland, New Jersey. I liked the idea of connecting the goats to my extended family; I already had a venerable ewe, an excellent mother, named Paula. I also thought Paula (the human one) would like goats — her kind of farm animal, useful and sensibly sized.

Sandy asked if I'd consider taking Honey as well. I said I'd think about it.

So Ruth and Murray were in residence — and spent their first two nights wailing for their mommy. I'd learned from my sheep that the connection between young animals and their mothers is strong, though transitory. They'd get over the loss, and food and shelter would go a long way toward comforting them.

Sandy and Keith had brought along a small wooden shelter, but the HBO Memorial Lambing Pen utterly overshadowed it. Sandy, a bit stunned, said it was the most beautiful goat house she'd ever seen.

After two days of piteous bleating, Ruth and Murray took to the farm — and why not? They had an acre of scrub to chew on. Annie was cooing to them and bringing them apple wafers and homemade grain treats. Paula, there for their arrival, plied them with stale Cheerios. I soon learned that they appreciated the microwaved popcorn leftovers from the night before.

I liked the way Murray and Ruth were always thoughtfully chewing on something. I liked their alertness and curiosity. I even appreciated the running commentary they offered every time I came outside. They were quick to run up to the fence, rest their hooves on the wire mesh, and jeer at me, a loud, nasal *maah* that was presumptuous and impertinent. They weren't reserved, either; they were the cable talk-show panelists of the animal world. I took to jeering back. "Nuts to you, goats! Bug off!"

It wasn't unusual to come out and see Murray or Ruth standing on the picnic table, or balancing atop the doghouse. They did escape almost at will, spotting tiny apertures I never noticed until I came outside and found them strolling around the back of the house. But they never went far from each other, their scrubby weeds, and their spectacular pen. They're not stupid, goats.

I'm not proud of the fact I was exchanging insults — most unfit for a family audience — with these imperious little creatures, but there it was.

I admit that I loved their insouciance, their authority issues, their rapt fascination with almost everything. Amid all these animals that revered me for bringing them food, it was refreshing to have a few who regularly taunted the hand that fed them.

I was happy to have them on my farm. A week later Sandy e-mailed to ask me about Honey, now that I knew what the others were like. The Adamses loved their goats, but for farmers, there's a hard point where reality and sentimentality clash.

Sure, I said. Bring her on over.

Yet goats can't really be the antidote to gloominess. Everyone around me was still warning that I seemed worn, joyless, dispirited. And they were right: I was starting to feel like a milk carton with a leak in the bottom; I didn't have much left.

I didn't really know why I was feeling so low. But when I grew tired, or discouraged, I did tend to drift toward my farm animals. Their existence can't really lift me up, but their very obliviousness to human emotions is comforting, somehow. Dogs can be sensitive to their owners' psyches; Izzy and Rose certainly are. Cows, on the other hand, don't really know or care about my moods. They stay steady in the face of human frailty, affectionate and focused on the apples or candy bars I'm carrying.

So the first living creature to whom I confided my problem was Elvis, my twenty-five-hundred-pound Brown Swiss steer.

Elvis was probably the only animal on the farm, with the exception of the dogs, who preferred to see me, rather than Annie, approaching. During his two years in residence, we'd bonded over a steady stream of apples, carrots, Snickers bars, and, throughout late summer, cornstalks. He loved cornstalks.

Elvis was the first animal in more than forty years that my dairy farmer friend Peter Hanks couldn't bear to send to market. He told me the gregarious steer followed him around the barn, stared at him, tried to lick him, and wouldn't walk onto the truck to the slaughterhouse.

When Peter considered who, among the people he knew with pastureland, was crazy enough to take in the steer he called "Brownie" and feed him for the rest of his life, he didn't come up with a long list of candidates. I went over to see the steer, who seemed nearly two stories tall, and bought him for $500. He was soon joined by Harold, another steer in need of adoption, and Luna, a mixed-breed cow.

Peter was right about this animal, whom I quickly renamed after the King. He had enormous brown eyes, and an unusual interest in people. Bigger than he realized, he could be inappropriately social, as in the morning he ambled over, picked me up by the hood of my sweatshirt, and dangled me happily for a few seconds, until I reached over and slugged him on the nose and he dropped me with a thud, looking surprised and hurt.

If he was grazing on the hilltop when I went out to the pasture in the morning, he would come thundering down the hill; I'd look up at this charging monster and dive behind a tree, since he couldn't stop for quite a while. Sometimes, in ice or mud, he had trouble stopping at all; I could imagine him shooting through the electrified fence and landing on a passing pickup.

He loved to drool on me, to rake his giant tongue across my shirt, or, better yet, the top of my head; he liked to eat my baseball caps.

In return, I scratched his neck and forehead while he closed his eyes in delight. I sprayed repellent on his face to try to keep the flies away, and rubbed balm on his scratches and sores.

There was something infectious about his sense of contentment — or I hoped there would be. I imagined him up on the hill, having spent his first two years inside a concrete-floored barn, contemplating the less fortunate cows we could see in the farms across in the valley.

Elvis was the picture of stability, equanimity, and even-temperedness, the polar opposite of the many excitable and dramatic people among whom I was raised. He offered the additional benefit of being unable to talk back.

So, early one fall morning, as Elvis lay splayed at the top of the pasture, munching on the remnants of a bag of carrots I'd brought, staring at me contentedly — he always reminded me of Shrek, the ugly but good-hearted ogre of literature and film — I decided to level with him. It seemed easier, somehow, to be honest with a steer.

"Dude," I said, sitting next to this mountain of a living thing, "I'm having trouble. I think I've slipped into the shadows, and I have to get out."

I told Elvis I needed spiritual renewal. I had lost perspective, wasn't enjoying much of anything. I needed to pay more attention to my family, my farm, my dogs and animals, my work, my friends. I needed faith — not necessarily the religious kind, but the belief and conviction that I could feel happy and optimistic again.

Elvis seemed to acknowledge my ideas, even approve of them, chewing thoughtfully, drooling plentifully, unruffled by the news.

I called Izzy, who'd been waiting and watching, and we began the long trek back down the hill. Elvis isn't like a dog; he didn't get up and follow me. He didn't need me to sit with him. He could be fond of me, at times, but could take me or leave, an easy relationship to have. I waved and said, "Thanks for listening."

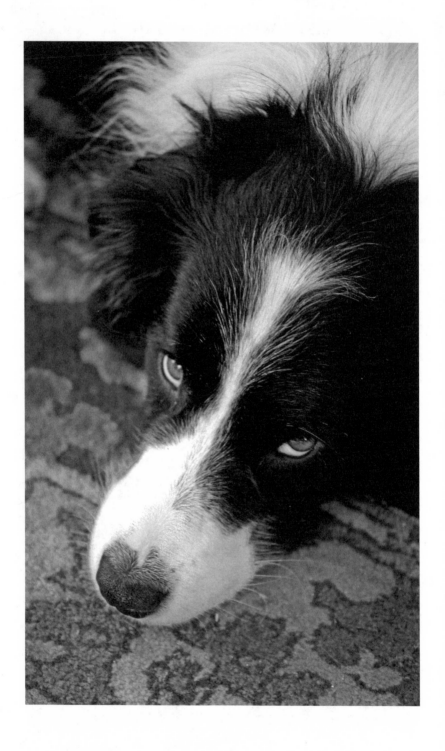

CHAPTER FIVE:
THE FARM WIFE

The hospice form dropped off at my house said that Etta was eighty-four, had lived all her life on a family farm, had been suffering from dementia and was now dying from colon cancer.

She'd been enrolled in hospice recently, which meant her doctors thought she had less than six months to live. We would find her in a nursing home in Granville, a poor, working-class town where decaying miners' houses alternated with equally decaying Victorians, and where dollar stores and bars were the liveliest businesses.

Etta's husband had died years ago, and a grandson and granddaughter out West were her only living relatives. She had no friends left alive who could visit her, no local relatives who could take her into their homes; given her medical condition, that might not even have been possible.

At the nursing home, Izzy and I were to

meet her grandson, Peter, in for a visit from Colorado. Etta's forms warned that she was medicated for severe pain, was no longer able to see or hear well, was subject to spells of panic.

She had owned many dogs in her years of farming, though, and was fond of them. The hope was that Izzy might calm her, making it easier to bathe, feed, and medicate her. The hospice philosophy called for her to be kept as comfortable as possible, and for her final days to be meaningful, even enjoyable. Frightened and confused by people, maybe she would respond to an animal.

I braced myself a bit; nursing homes were tough places. In private homes, there were usually family members around, a loving and supportive atmosphere. Patients drew considerable comfort from being around their loved ones, in familiar surroundings.

Institutions were another story. Nursing homes were chronically short-staffed, the patients often alone in their rooms much of the day. Sometimes there was family around, or friends; often not.

The homes I'd seen were depressing, dimly lit, and cheerless despite the piped-in music and silk flowers placed strategically on tables and bedstands.

Beyond that, the ambivalence in these

places about hospice workers and volunteers was noticeable. Hospice offers a choice, a way to die — without invasive procedures, emergency hospital visits, the dramatic and artificial prolonging of life. In health-care facilities, and even among some family members, calling in hospice is seen as giving up, surrendering to death rather than nobly fighting it.

The middle-aged son of one dying woman took me aside as Izzy and I were preparing to enter the house. He wanted to be sure I understood where he stood. "Look, I know you're trying to do good, but to me you're the angel of death," he said, almost angrily. "We're not going to quit. My mom is going to make it. She's a fighter, she's gonna hang in there." Three weeks later, she died, and I wondered how much her son might have left unsaid.

In nursing homes, I sometimes picked up this uneasy vibe from the staff. They were intent on keeping their patients alive, not helping them to die. It showed up in subtle ways — a cool greeting, quiet comments. All in all, going into nursing homes felt different from seeing people in their own homes. But that made it all the more important to go, because these patients might be even more alone.

The cold, raw, drizzly November day didn't help. Izzy jumped out of the car, checking out the parking lot with that eager-to-go-to-work border collie look. I leashed him up, as regulations required, and affixed our ID tags, and we headed into the lobby.

Two or three elderly women in wheelchairs were delighted to see us, and Izzy went over to each of them, so they could pat him and reminisce about their own pets. I was struck anew at how much pleasure he gave people, just by his presence, the way he greeted each person individually. He always made eye contact, always waited patiently and happily for a hug or a scratch, and he'd learned to listen attentively to stories about Buddy or Duke. These memories, of beloved though long-gone dogs, seemed to open people up, put them in touch with a warmer, happier part of their lives.

This nursing home was a modern brick-and-stucco structure that looked clean and colorful. Maybe, you wanted to think, people lived well here. Yet there was not much activity. The patients — mostly older women — sat around tables or on benches, some gazing at a television set, others keeping an eye on the lobby traffic. Although Thanksgiving had not yet come, Christmas music was already wafting from the speakers.

"Oh, I wish he could live here," said one woman, talking more to Izzy than to me. "But I wouldn't wish that on him. I'm sure he's happy where he is."

We checked in with the manager, who said hello, looked indifferently at Izzy — no pats or hugs here — and led us down a long hallway. Etta's grandson was already in the room, we were told en route. He had flown in for a day or so. But apart from him and the hospice social workers and nursing staff, Etta had had no visitors.

The manager opened a door at the end of the corridor, showed us in without comment, and left.

The room was warm and clean, with a cluster of family photos — kids, a baby, holiday dinners, and, yes, a dog — placed around the dresser, along with china figurines.

Peter, a fit, middle-aged man in elaborate cowboy boots, was sitting on the bed, looking uncomfortable. Colorado must have seemed a long way off.

Across from him, sitting in a green upholstered chair, was a frail-looking woman in a nightgown that was pulled up to her thighs. A crocheted afghan sat balled up on the floor by her feet. She was clutching her side. "Sit down, sit down," she moaned.

"I don't know what to do," the young man said distractedly, as we entered the room. "She's agitated. She keeps throwing that afghan off. And I think she's in pain." I took Izzy off the leash; tail swishing, he walked straight to Peter, who looked relieved to see him. Perhaps he was relieved to see anyone.

Then Izzy saw Etta, and seemed to refocus, get serious. He turned toward her, approaching slowly, resting his head on her exposed knee. One hand twisted her nightgown; with the other, she held her side. She seemed unaware of the dog.

Suddenly, she let out a cry and hit Izzy sharply across the nose with the back of her hand, swatting at him, shouting out, "Get away! Get on the floor!" Izzy, startled, backed away quickly, turning to me. I had him lie down.

We'd been trained for this, to encounter hostility and pretend it hadn't happened. Expect anything, we'd been told a hundred times; by now we did.

"Hello, Etta," I said. "I'm Jon and this is Izzy. We came to visit you. I know you had dogs on your farm and loved dogs, so we thought we would just spend a few minutes here with you, if that's okay."

In hospice, one of the first things you learn is to talk to people who are not necessarily talking back, who may not seem to even hear you. Some patients are perfectly lucid and some, like Etta, suffer dementia and move in and out of reality. You never really know for sure what someone's mental state is, so you just carry on as if the conversation is flowing normally and hope some of your message, or just the sound of your voice, filters through.

After a while, it doesn't matter what the patients say, you realize. What matters is that a conversation takes place, even a one-sided one, that there's some connection. Communication is a fluid thing when it comes to those at the end of their lives.

But it's not an easy thing to do, having that sort of conversation. It goes against the grain of normal interaction, and requires you to be up, attentive, and enthusiastic, whether or not you're getting anything back. And Izzy was used to appreciation and affection, not rejection. He looked a bit perplexed. This wasn't the usual script.

He waited a couple of minutes, then drifted back to Etta. She startled, lashed out again, swatting at his head, but this time he was ready and quickly backed out of range, looking confused.

I called him off to regroup and try to figure things out. I thought conversation might be best.

Peter and I both talked to Etta for a bit, asking how she was, if she was in pain, if she needed anything. She seemed restless, leaning over, clutching her side, fidgeting with her nightgown, rocking back and forth. Sometimes she said something I could understand — "Sit down, sit down" — and at other times her sounds were wordless.

I wasn't sure if we ought to continue the visit, or perhaps come again another day. Yet the hospice nurses, who wanted Etta to be more comfortable if at all possible, had urged me to come with Izzy.

By now, a couple of months into hospice work, Izzy was developing instincts of his own, picking up confidence along the way. He experienced these visits as his work, I'd come to see, in the same way Rose looked forward to herding sheep. I could see how he enjoyed being successful, getting praise, connecting with people.

Usually he went right to the patient, in a bed or chair. He was becoming skilled at navigating rooms crowded with wheelchairs, hospital beds, oxygen tanks, people in close quarters.

His border collie agility came in handy — in one home he had to hop onto a bed that was a virtual minefield of medical equipment. When it was time for him to jump off,

I held my breath; how could he fail to entangle himself in the IV tubes or collide with the commode or hit the patient's foot? But he moved delicately, threading the needle, with no problem. My trust in him in these situations was growing.

Our conversation having no apparent effect, Peter gestured for me to come into the hallway with him. "I love my grandmother, but I just can't take it anymore, seeing her like this," he confessed. "She doesn't know me and I'm not helping her. I always remember her on the farm, with her dogs, busy and hospitable, baking pies and cookies, always happy and so full of life. I can't handle this right now. I'm grateful to you for coming, but do you mind if I wait outside?"

I told him I understood. Sometimes, it's just too much. Sometimes, when you are watching people you love move toward death, you do have to step outside. I decided to keep trying. Rather, Izzy decided for me.

When I returned, I saw that he had quietly approached Etta again, from a different angle. He came to the hand she held at her side, slowly wriggled his nose beneath it, and sat still.

She looked surprised. "Oh," she said. "A dog. There's a dog." She took a deep breath, said something I couldn't decipher, then looked down at Izzy. She seemed to be struggling to piece things together — the strangers, the dog, her anxiety. Her face, drawn and ashen, looked different, her features rearranging themselves. I saw a hint of a smile, or thought I did.

"I'm so sorry," she said, quaveringly but distinctly now. "So sorry. No biscuits, no tea, no place to sit. A dog!" Something, some memory, had pulled her out of herself. Without question, she looked more comfortable. Peter, watching from the hall, came and stood in the doorway. How strange, I thought, for Izzy, Etta, and me to be together in this room, this place, at this time.

"God, I haven't yet seen her smile," Peter said, stunned. So he'd seen it, too. "I didn't think she could anymore."

As Izzy sat motionless, Etta moved her hand along his slender nose, rubbed his forehead.

Less fearful, she was regaining some dignity, the person she was — is — becoming visible through her confusion and discomfort. This was a woman used to taking care of guests, offering them homemade pie, making sure they were comfortable. Maybe that's why she'd been asking us to sit down.

Now she was apologizing, apparently, because she couldn't give us food or tea. Peter and I reassured her that she didn't have to worry about that, that we understood.

Peter picked up the afghan and tucked it over her knees, and she allowed him to. Her hand on Izzy's head, she stopped clutching her side. The smile on her face expanded a little. Her mouth moved, but now no words emerged that we could understand.

Peter went to find an aide, who appeared in a few minutes and looked surprised. "I don't think I've seen her smile before," she said. She called for another aide to help.

While Izzy and I stepped outside, they got Etta up, sponge-bathed and changed her, and got her into bed, arranging a bright quilt over her.

When I came back inside, she was moaning softly, talking, but her demeanor was much easier, her face more peaceful. In a few minutes, she fell asleep.

Izzy came over to the bed and rested his head next to her hand, but she was no longer aware of any of us. "Okay, Izzy, that'll do," I said, the command used to tell a border collie his work was finished.

So he went over to nuzzle Peter, and then the slightly taken-aback aides. "Good dog, Izzy," one said, then quickly went into the bathroom to wash her hands.

It took us nearly an hour to get back down

the corridor and through the lobby, past Izzy's many new fans and admirers. Spotting one tiny woman half-dozing in her wheelchair, one leg dangling down to the footrest, the other amputated at the knee, Izzy walked over to gently lay his head on the bandaged stump.

"My, my," the woman said, noticing her visitor. "Where on earth did you come from, you handsome thing?"

CHAPTER SIX:
LENORE

The puppy was just past six weeks old and was marching right through a tub of mushy dog food, scarfing it up as she went, when she looked up and saw me standing outside the kennel fence. She was jet black, pudgy, with a bit of attitude. Her alert eyes focused on me, on her hungry littermates, on the food bowl. Then she yawned, wagged, and went back to her meal.

Labrador retrievers, even very young ones, keep their priorities straight: no mission trumps eating.

This one, a female, caught my eye from the first. She was already a beautiful dog with a classic square head and body and jet-black eyes full of mischief.

Two of her siblings were throwing themselves against the fence, trying to attract my attention, and two barely seemed to notice me at all. This one had a take-it-or-leave-it stance that I looked for in puppies — inter-

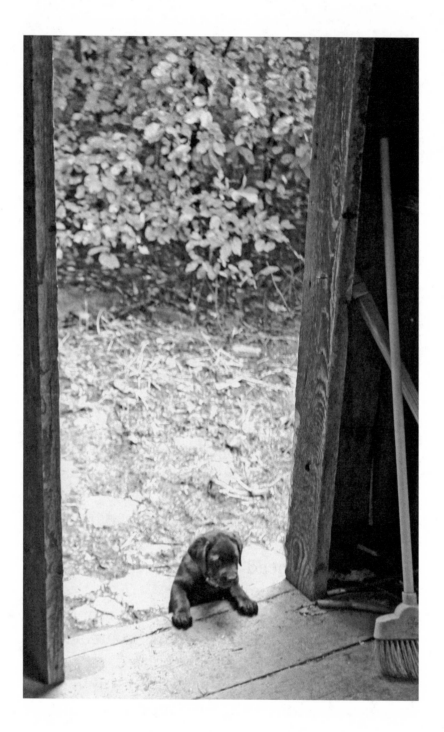

ested but neither too excited nor too stand-
offish.

I was interested, too.

The e-mail, from Gretchen Pinkel of Kee-
Pin Labs in neighboring Argyle, had announced the arrival of a new litter. I know a
lot of breeders and I often get birth an-
nouncements. People warn that it's dangerous to go see a puppy if you're not looking
for one, but I was rarely tempted to bring
one home. I hadn't raised a puppy for several
years. I just like meeting breeders: seeing
their Labs, poodles, shepherds, border collies; sitting around and yakking about dogs,
dog lovers, breeds, trials, and training. Nobody knows more about canines or enjoys
talking about them more; I always learn
something.

I'd met Gretchen at a book reading, and
around town. She and her husband, John,
for whom dogs were clearly a passion, had a
contemporary house, with part of their yard
devoted to kennels. Gretchen was also a conscientious breeder, choosing bitches and
sires carefully, hauling her dogs to trials and
shows, reading books and talking to vets. But
she and John also just plain liked dogs; you
could tell by the stories they told about their
dogs, by their humor and great tolerance for

Lab behaviors, like eating revolting things, then vomiting them up all over the house.

From time to time, I drove over to Argyle and sat outside with them. Gretchen and John were always hospitable, pulling out a few lawn chairs, some local cider and corn muffins, and chatting easily.

The travails of breeding are many: coping with health issues, competing and showing, choosing which dog to breed and supervising the tricky birthing process, then anxiously evaluating how things have gone and looking for good homes for the newcomers. It's not easy to breed well.

Like most good breeders, Gretchen was a bit obsessive about matching puppies up with the right owners. Along with all they know about canine genetics and temperaments, breeders often prove to be keen evaluators of human psychology. Gretchen and John stayed up nights fussing over whether this dog would suit that person, trying to divine from afar the human's personality and patience and training notions.

It was always in the air that I might be interested in one of their Labs one day, but I also made it clear that my life was hectic and that I wasn't currently in the market. That was fine with Gretchen and John; good breeders don't want their dogs going to anybody who isn't completely sure.

Dog lovers always want a dog, of course, and continually grapple with the impulsive desire to have one more. I feel it, too, at times.

And while there are all kinds of ways to acquire a great dog — shelters, rescue groups, breeders — and I've loved my rescued dogs, I have to admit my favorite method is to let a good breeder help me choose one.

But when Gretchen's e-mail announced that the newest puppies had arrived, I told her I wasn't ready for a new dog at the moment. Still, I'd love to come by and see them.

It had been a challenging few months. After spending most of the summer and into the fall on a book tour, filled with warm, appreciative readers but also with delayed planes, many hours in airport lounges and in cars, and lunches of low-carb snack bars, I already felt spent. And always, there was the farm. I did not, I told myself, want a dog now.

The past year had gotten so frantic I'd allowed my daughter to take Pearl, my sweet-tempered senior dog, to live with her in Brooklyn, where she was thriving. My other yellow Lab, Clementine, was living most of the time in Vermont with my former physical therapist, who had the time and energy to take her into the woods for hikes, to lakes for swims, for mountain treks I couldn't match.

Having let go of two Labs I cherished, why would I acquire another when I was arguably even busier? For most of the year, I thought it a bad idea. But I do love the companionship of dogs, and I do love acquiring them carefully and training them thoughtfully. Much to my surprise, and thanks to the help of many others, I've become pretty good at it. Somehow, the trials of the past year had caused me to lose touch with that part of myself. I wanted to reconnect with it.

Plus, I was down one dog. For much of the year, I'd enjoyed the company of, and conversation with, Emma, the lovable border collie who'd shared the same fenced enclosure as Izzy. She came to me after problems developed in her other home. Emma was older than Izzy and riddled with health problems — Lyme disease, heartworms, kidney trouble — so I'd promised I'd get her well and stable, then find a good home for her.

I loved having Emma here, throatily grumbling and murmuring to me while I was working, but I'd always planned to re-home her. The farm was too active, even chaotic, for her; she fled at the sight of sheep and couldn't run alongside my ATV with Rose and Iz. What she needed was a quieter place, ideally one with a sheepskin rug thrown over a sofa or chair for her comfort. All she really wanted was to nap and be cuddled, and she deserved that.

My philosophy, which I know distresses some dog lovers, is that it can be okay — it can sometimes be wonderful, in fact — to bring dogs home, treat their problems, train them lovingly, and then find congenial homes that make the dogs and other humans happy. I operate a sort of unofficial placement service that has given me and others a lot of pleasure. While some think it's heresy to ever give a dog you love away, I find it can be immensely satisfying.

Still, when a dog who's been here a while does leave — I had found a sweet family nearby for gentle Emma, one able to monitor her health care — it always leaves me with a bit of an ache.

So I had an opening on the farm and in my psyche. I was thinking about a working dog, a dog bred to do things with humans, to go places, a dog who might lift me up and get me focused again. I had two border collies, and no sane person wants three border collies.

I wanted a dog that might be able to do

hospice work like Izzy, that could safely visit a school or a mall, or go along on a book tour and lie happily at my feet while I talked. My dogs have to handle a lot of challenges, so temperament, a cornerstone of any good breeding program, was critical. I wanted another Lab.

This little black pup, I have to say, touched something in me. I told John and Gretchen that I would like to come back in a couple of days. They nodded politely — responsible breeders never push anybody to get a dog — and said I would be welcome. I said I'd bring Rose and Izzy along.

I knew I was in trouble when I mentioned the puppy to a friend. She suggested a name — Lenore — from Edgar Allan Poe's "The Raven." I knew from past experience that when you name a puppy, you're already making a commitment. I called Paula in New Jersey and told her I had met a puppy.

"Did you give it a name?" she asked warily.

"Yes," I said. "Lenore."

Her sigh could be heard half a mile away.

On my third visit to see Lenore, she had evolved, as puppies do as they approach their eighth week. Gretchen pulled out the lawn chairs and the muffins.

Earlier, Lenore had given me the eye, permitted me a few pats, happily accepting a

112

tiny biscuit. Izzy and Rose had sniffed her perfunctorily, then ignored her.

This time she spotted me right away and came over to the fence, wagging her tail. She was beginning to recognize me. Gretchen put her in my lap and she settled, as if she'd been there before, quite comfortably and naturally. She leaned her head against my chest and went to sleep.

Gretchen and John exchanged glances. "We've read your books, and this is the dog we thought you might choose," she said. "When you said you were coming over to see the litter, we didn't know if you would take one or not. And it's fine if you don't. But we both thought this dog would be great for you. She's sweet and calm, nice disposition. And she's going to be beautiful."

All true.

I had Googled Poe's poem, so I pulled a copy from my shirt pocket and read a verse or two aloud: "It shall clasp a sainted maiden whom the angels name Lenore — / Clasp a rare and radiant maiden whom the angels name Lenore . . ." Gretchen looked a bit startled, but smiled. Lenore yawned and, unmoved, went back to sleep.

This puppy had perspective, I thought. She was contemplative. She had soul. She was a Lab.

That night, I drove to PetSmart, bought yet another crate, a couple of bags of rawhide and training treats, a tiny collar — and lots of odor repellent and disinfectant.

I was excited, eager to get to know this pup. She had the potential, I felt, of becoming one of those patient, affectionate dogs you could take anywhere, a dog that could, if properly trained and socialized and acclimated, move freely among humans, not have to be walled off from them.

I treasure my border collies and the extraordinary things they can do. Herding sheep with Rose, making visits with Izzy, it's been rewarding almost beyond my imagination. Still, when people ask me what the best all-around breed is, pound for pound, I never hesitate to say it's a Lab. One of the best working dogs, one of the best family dogs, one of the best dogs, period.

And yet, like some other popular breeds, the Labrador has suffered profoundly from commercialization. Once too many families wanted Labs, proliferating puppy mills and careless, indifferent breeders created far too many of them, with scant attention to health and temperament. The relentless drive of the market can, in a blink, nearly obliterate a breed's best traits. Then the impulsive and thoughtless way many people get dogs, the

114

lack of dog training, aggravates the problem.

Labs have been bred for centuries to be with humans, to work with us, to be calm and patient. Yet the image of the goofy, over-enthusiastic Labrador, jumping up on people, snatching food out of their hands, ravaging kitchen cabinets and garbage cans, has become commonplace — and deservedly so.

But that's a disservice to their proud heritage. I've had a series of great Labs from good breeders, so I see them differently. They're tolerant, calm, genial, responsive, eager to please. From puppyhood, they know almost everything they need to know — except how to be calm. One of the joys of my life as a dog owner is showing border collies and Labs how to chill, to fit into my routine, not disrupt it, to live up to their storied potential as humans' partners, not lunging, hyperkinetic creatures to be incessantly scolded and chided.

Just thinking about this process made me look forward to an autumn with Lenore, recharging my passion for good dogs, for showing them how to live in our world.

I started counting the days — six — until she could leave her litter and come to the farm. When I got home, I sat down with a notebook, jotted some reminders for myself, and reviewed my training philosophy —

what I'd learned, what had worked and what hadn't. Lenore seemed a dog that could be all the things I wanted, if I didn't mess her up.

On my latest visit, I'd told her of my ambitions. "I want you to be calm and easy," I said as she gnawed on my chin. "I want you to go places with me, to know almost every kind of person, to hear car horns and sirens and coyote howls without getting scared or going nuts. You'll be gentle with kids, appropriate with older people, good around other dogs. I don't want you running off, either." She stopped chewing and licked me; maybe I was getting through already.

Smiling down at this affectionate, attentive creature, I realized that getting Lenore was already lifting my fatigue, brightening my funk, reminding me why I was up here in the country, and what I loved.

Back in Bedlam, she was curious and relentlessly affectionate; she stayed close. The first two nights, she yowled and shrieked downstairs in her crate, undoubtedly missing her mom and littermates. The din was unholy, and both Rose and Izzy retreated upstairs with me and hid under the bed.

It was a battle I couldn't lose, and I didn't. The third night Lenore went into the crate, fell asleep, and was quiet all night. I reinforced the idea of the crate as a safe, comforting place by hand-feeding her inside it sometimes, and by tossing in some kibble so she would always find goodies there when I yelled "Crate! Crate!" I stocked it with toys and chewbones, too, so she would associate the crate with fun.

Her fellow canines were another matter. Border collies can be humorless and contemptuous. Rose, who doesn't really grasp the concept of play, growled and nipped at the newcomer, or ran from her. Izzy pretended not to notice she was there. Lenore, undeterred, approached the other two, gnawed on their ruffs, licked them. No dice. Once, she tried to share the bone Rose was chewing on: I heard a sudden growl and a shriek, and Lenore came catapulting toward me and hid between my legs. Game over.

Outdoors, she ran up to greet the goats, but all three took off for the far side of their pen. A new dog required some adjustment. The donkeys lowered their ears and backed away; Mother and Minnie, the barn cats, vanished.

It was left to Elvis to appreciate this little dog. He was the only resident, besides me, unequivocally happy to see her, perhaps because they shared profoundly sweet natures.

It was striking to see this little black pup, not yet much bigger than my hand, rush out to visit the enormous steer, her tail swinging.

I kept her on a leash, prepared to pluck her up off the ground if there was any trouble. But Elvis just widened his enormous brown eyes, lowered his great head, and sneezed, covering her in drooly gook. A true Lab, she appreciated that and wriggled over to lick him on the nose.

Day by day, she persisted in her getting-to-know-you campaign. The goats, curious by nature, watched her from a distance, and then, after a few days, began rushing up to the fence to greet her. The barn cats may never appreciate her rushing at them, but at least they stopped fleeing at the sight of her. Even Winston the rooster continued pecking at grubs and worms while Lenore ran circles around him.

As for me, the first night, I plucked Lenore off the floor and tucked her on the sofa next to me, to doze and cuddle there while I read.

Hand-feeding was a good strategy; it meant Lenore paid close attention to me and my hands. Her name recognition, already good, was greatly enhanced by the judicious application of some liver treats, tossed on the ground while I called her name. She was a quick study. After she ate, she went into the crate; forty-five minutes later, I walked her outside on a leash and she did her business and got praise and another liver treat. She was mostly housebroken in less than a week.

But the most fun part of having a puppy — any puppy, but especially a Lab — is seeing their impact on people. Too bad I didn't know until midlife the heady impact puppies have on women of all ages; to call Lenore a chick magnet is an understatement. Women pulled over in their cars, came running out of stores, or rushed across parking lots to see Lenore, to bury their faces in her sleek black fur, to croon "Awwww, puppy!" and "How adorable!"

They ask Lenore's name, beg to hold her, ask her age and where she came from. They don't ask *my* name, or exclaim over my cuteness, but I'm happy to bask in Lenore's reflected glory.

And not only women were smitten. Annie's gruff husband, Joe, who has refused for years to get a dog, preferring the company of goats and a rabbit, melted like an ice cube in July when he saw Lenore. He invited her for sleepovers. (I agreed, until she got into their goat pen and also started sampling the rabbit food, resulting in my going through a quart of odor repellent in two days.)

Lenore is a portable happiness generator,

triggering smiles and exclamations, leavings oohs and aahs in her wake. Neighbors drove several miles to see her. One brought her ailing grandmother, just to gaze out the car window and see Lenore, and I could hear their joyous exclamations from inside the farmhouse. The UPS driver threatened to steal her.

If Rose's work ethic dominated the farm, and Izzy was my shadow and companion, Lenore was light itself, suffusing the place with affection.

I can't look at her without smiling. When Izzy and I dragged ourselves home from a hospice visit, Lenore came bounding, almost exploding with joy when she saw us. Lenore's big heart and good nature could pierce armor. They certainly pierced mine. I love all my dogs, but I could not remember being so smitten by a puppy. Yet no matter how excited she got, when I picked her up, she put her head on my shoulder, calmed down, and went to sleep.

And I made sure to spread her cheer. I took the business of canine socialization seriously, and if ever a dog was ready to learn to be social, it was Lenore.

I toted her to the gas station. To Gardenworks. To the dentist and the post office. Down Main Street in Salem, to the mall in

Saratoga, and the supermarket parking lot in Greenwich. Lines of people, mostly women, formed to cuddle her and kiss her on the nose.

I had my standards. I'd told Gretchen that Lenore would spend the night in her crate for six months, at least, before she was permitted to sleep in a place of her own choosing. After many wrestling matches in bed over the years with burrowed-in snoring Labs, I decreed that this dog would be crated until she was no longer a puppy. There's no reason for young dogs to sleep outside a crate; they can only get into trouble. They're just as happy to be in a crate — especially one lined in fleece and stuffed with toys and bones — as out, and I am happier.

Lenore accepted this regimen, although when I headed upstairs at night, I'd sometimes hear a whimper from her crate.

About eight weeks after Lenore arrived, the first real cold snap of the winter hit. Cold spells upstate frequently involve howling winds and temperatures plunging well below zero. The old farmhouse was rattling; the donkeys and sheep had retreated into the pole barn.

I tossed a biscuit into Lenore's crate and

said, "Yo! Crate!" and she trotted in as always, looking for the treat she by now knew to expect. Then she pressed her small head against the closing gate. I thought I saw her shiver; I definitely heard a single plaintive yelp.

"Maybe just this one awful night," I said, reopening the gate and reaching for her as she wriggled happily into my arms. A few minutes later, she was nestled contentedly against the small of my back and I couldn't turn over for fear of mashing her. So I slept on my side, happily, all through that long and cold night. Most nights, now, Lenore, to my wife's displeasure, has taken up residence.

I'll regret this, perhaps, as Lenore grows bigger. Much bigger. But for now, on bitter winter nights, she curls against me and keeps my back warm, and the sound of her melodic snoring fuses with Winston's persistent crowing to create a sweet farm symphony.

CHAPTER SEVEN: INTO THE WOODS

On my first extended trek into the wild, I looked at my trail map, studied it carefully, and turned left when I should have gone right. My friend Anthony, with his dog Mo and daughter Ida in tow, looked at me doubtfully, but — as I was the navigator — followed my lead.

The Merck Forest, in western Vermont, encompasses three thousand acres of mountains, hills, valleys, and deep forest. I'd hiked here many times with my dogs, but this would be my first overnight. It was late fall, the afternoon sunshine strong, but the already chilling nights were a sharp reminder of the winter coming.

Several hours later, as the sky was darkening and the temperature starting to plummet, we all staggered into the clearing around the rustic cabin I'd reserved. I marveled that I'd made it. It was supposed to be a two-mile trek to this spot, but my error had

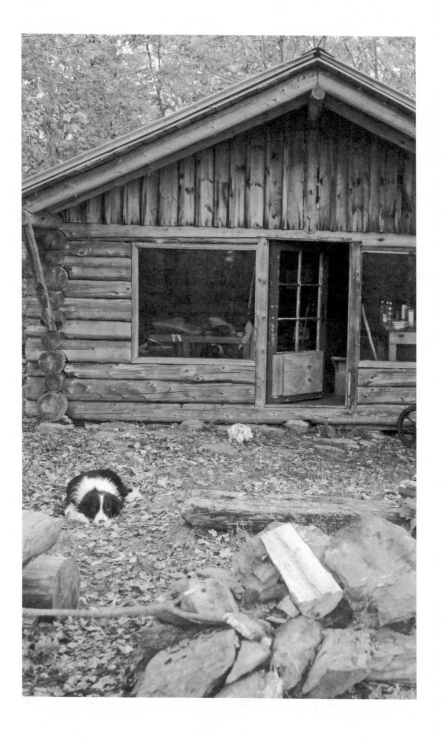

probably made it much longer. Twice, Anthony had taken my backpack and hoisted it himself, along with his own. Even Izzy, fit and lean, collapsed on the cabin floor and passed out.

Fortunately, we'd left early enough to reach the cabin with some daylight remaining. But we'd left some of the heavier equipment behind on the trail, and Anthony hiked back to retrieve it.

The place was almost instantly worth it, though. A three-quarter moon popped up in the valley below, and some giant owls — I could see only their silhouettes in the moonlight, and their vast eyes — settled in the trees in front of the cabin to hoot and stare. The wind rustled the few leaves remaining on the trees.

A great soothing calm descended on us.

The mechanics of camping are daunting, especially for a disorganized, clumsy novice like me. Backpacks are no longer simple canvas-and-buckle affairs but elaborate high-tech mechanisms with space-age frames, involving weight-bearing strategies and various secret compartments.

Food isn't simple, either. If the weather is warm, you need a cooler, and if you need a cooler, you need a big person to tote it in. If the weather is cold, you can hang food on a hook outside the cabin and it will stay fresh — but then you need ways to keep yourself warm.

The cabin was a simple wooden structure, the size of a small living room, with a wood-stove at its center. Its previous occupants had put out the fire, cleaned out the cabin, and left behind a jug of water and a roll of toilet paper, as camping etiquette dictated; I made a note to always do the same.

I'd come to Merck hoping for a sense of spiritual renewal. Something was wrong with me and I knew it, so I decided to try some things I'd never done. The solitude of the woods might help, I thought. I would climb out of my familiar environment, spend time someplace where I might see myself more clearly, and begin what I already suspected was going to be a lengthy process of questioning, thinking, and changing. I wanted to be refreshed.

We sat out by a campfire, eating the chicken dinner Anthony prepared. He and Ida would spend the night, and then they would hike out; other friends would come and help me backpack out.

It was humbling, even painful, to realize that camping was not something I could do by myself. I could sit by a fire, read and stare and take photos. But I was no longer physically up to hauling stuff miles into the woods alone. My bad ankle protested the hills, and I knew my back would have something to say about sleeping on wooden boards in the cold.

As a general rule, I don't do things I can't handle myself, so this dependence was difficult to acknowledge.

But I'd slowly come to realize that I couldn't run the farm by myself any longer, either, not like I had the first couple of years, hauling hay bales, moving firewood, walking across the ice to reposition feeders and drag water hoses and grain buckets. I wasn't old, but I wasn't young, either, and the farm had taken a toll on my body.

I couldn't count the times I'd gone down on the ice, sometimes briefly losing consciousness, probably suffering a concussion or two. One day, my doctor warned, you will not wake up quickly and then you will be in trouble, especially in the cold. Or you will break something that can't easily be fixed.

Already I'd hit an unwelcome benchmark, the first chronic illness. In the spring, after bouts of fatigue and incessant running to the bathroom, I'd been diagnosed with diabetes. It shouldn't have come as a surprise, but I was stunned.

I've always proudly and stubbornly dismissed health nuts, dieters, food obsessives who take twenty minutes to order a meal in a restaurant. I had no desire to hang around doctors' offices or browse medical websites. I'd paid no attention to my weight in years. As a result I was quite overweight — and sick.

I did the change-your-lifestyle thing with a vengeance, largely forswearing desserts and bread; learning to read food labels; acquiring an endocrinologist and a nutritionist; becoming one of those people grilling waiters about sauces and salad dressings. I rode my ATV less and walked more. I lost more than fifty pounds and found that my back wasn't hurting so much and that I had more energy than I'd felt in years. My doctor was thrilled.

But it had been a challenging and chastening process, and now I was toting a lot of spinach, whole-grain bread, and my blood-glucose monitor into the woods with me.

I could have the farm, love it, and live on it; I could hike and even camp. But not without help.

It had only slowly occurred to me that I wasn't as strong or resilient as I'd been. I couldn't be as self-sufficient, couldn't help others the way I thought I could. It was occurring to me more this fall; in fact, it was being pounded into my skull.

I was getting it. I didn't like it.

I'd never gone camping before. But then I'd never run a farm before, never driven a tractor or cuddled with a twenty-five-hundred-pound steer. Maybe it was high time.

Camping always seemed one of those inexplicably uncomfortable things other people did — more fit and outdoorsy people. So I was amazed at how instantly I loved it, and how much more of it I wanted.

Still, it was a learning process of intimidating proportions. I'd come into the woods carrying about five times as much food as I needed, but not enough water for three people and two dogs. I'd brought books by C. S. Lewis and Thomas Merton, mysteries by Michael Connelly and James Lee Burke, Robert Frost's poetry. I carried my Canon 5-D camera with five different lenses and filter kits. I brought a half-gallon of milk, a box of Cheerios, a pack of turkey franks. Plus a couple of sweatshirts, two pairs of jeans, extra socks and underwear, three flashlights, and batteries.

Anthony cursed me roundly for packing all this stuff, and I have to admit I felt like a British viceroy on safari. I soon learned that you don't need a half-gallon of milk, for example, merely a packet of powdered milk to mix with water. You don't need an entire box of cereal, just two or three servings in a small bag. Bread and cheese and fruit will do nicely for a day or two; I didn't need elaborate meals.

Your sweatshirt can double as a pillow. One flannel shirt will do. You can't read four or five books; one will serve, preferably a paperback. Instead of a fully loaded camera bag, you can wear a camera around your neck and stash one additional lens in your backpack. You do need water, lots of it, and water is heavy.

Minimalism and simplicity don't come naturally to me, but I do learn. The second time I trekked into Merck, I would bring a third of what I'd brought this time.

Still, I was stunned at how much effort is required to spend a simple, quiet weekend in the mountains. The outhouse seemed a good quarter-mile away — though it was undoubtedly closer — and the woodshed even farther.

Every time I got settled, I had to get up and let the dogs out, prepare some food, get more firewood, or hike to the bathroom. It added up to a lot of walking and hauling.

My bunk was a few wooden boards. The

wind sliced right through the cabin walls at night, and I sorely regretted not stoking the fire even more. I learned quickly about the importance of matches and warm socks.

For Anthony, thirty and in great shape, camping was a hoot, almost instinctive. For me, at sixty, it represented moments of extraordinary peace and beauty interspersed with hours of frozen extremities, sleeplessness, and exhaustion. Yet being there was worth all that and more.

I appreciated Merck's beauty and majestic silence, but perhaps even more I appreciated being out of touch. Cell phones, iPods, e-mail, and pagers have nearly obliterated the experience of really being by yourself, of being able to hear yourself think. My friends usually think I'm in trouble if I don't return their calls in minutes, assuming that I'm always near some kind of communications device. Usually I am.

In the woods, I was truly incommunicado. Cell phones don't operate there even if you want to use them, and I didn't want to. There's no electricity, not to mention plumbing or heat. The only snazzy technology I had, besides my camera and the backpack frames, were LED flashlights — small, bright, made to last forever. Otherwise, it was just me and nature and the inside of my head.

And Izzy. Izzy loved being outdoors, though he wasn't inclined to overdo it. He appreciated walking with me a bit, but happily curled up underneath one of the bunk beds at night while I sat by the fire and read.

In fact, he was the perfect companion for a cramped cabin, with his genius for being nearly invisible in any room. When summoned to eat or hike, he appeared immediately; otherwise he made himself scarce, pursuing his own meditation. He did like sharing the bunk with me at night, though, as the wind rattled the cabin windows.

And he accompanied me on my first nocturnal trip to the outhouse, a drama that reinforced the new idea that on a camping expedition everything needs to be anticipated and planned for. If you wake up at three a.m., you'd better know where your glasses are, and your shoes, and your flashlight. Otherwise, you will step on a log or a dog or stub your toes or bang your head or stumble around in the dark.

In the outhouse, shivering and listening to the wind bluster outside the flimsy wooden door, you were led to unique reflection on the perils and benefits of modern life versus life as it used to be. I was glad Izzy had come along and sat pondering with me.

Still, it was lovely to sit under the open sky,

reading Merton's reflections on solitude by campfire light and flashlight. Ida was asleep inside, Anthony was reading on the other side of the fire, Izzy was draped by my feet. The clarity of the stars made it difficult to stay focused on the book.

In the morning, we toasted bread and wolfed down cereal. Anthony and Ida and Mo left, and I sat out in front of the cabin, watching the clouds sweep across the valley, soaking up the sounds of the birds conversing. I sat there for two hours. Took a walk, took some photos, read a book, then sat some more.

I loved the stillness, the absence of manmade noises, the sound of the air moving through the trees and across the meadows. This was a good place to take pictures, a good place to walk with my dog, a good place to think.

Seeking solitude can seem forced. Going off to Merck didn't necessarily mean I would have great insights, reach epiphanies, easily find renewal.

It was a tool, a new weapon in my arsenal. I suspected I was heading into the shadows, and was girding for what might be a long battle.

I went camping four times that fall and early winter. Sometimes Anthony walked me in, sometimes Bill and Maria, sometimes Maria by herself.

I was embarrassed to always need some help packing and hiking in and out; that alone marked a humbling need to accept a new reality.

When I look back on those excursions, I think of sitting by a campfire yakking with Anthony, or sitting and reading by myself in the dark cabin, warmed by the woodstove, the wind menacing outside. I think of long walks in the woods with Izzy, more light coming through the leafless trees with each trip, and of lying in wait with my camera for the sunrise, like a hunter stalking game.

I learned a bit more each time about how to pack, how to conserve water, how to make my bunk more comfortable. I tried to drink in the quiet and the peacefulness, as if I could bottle it and bring it back with me. Two or three times I was engulfed by loneliness and sadness. Once or twice, I felt waves of fear and inner darkness.

The last trip, late in November, was different from the others. Maria walked me in and helped me set up camp, but this stay never became settled or peaceful. I felt anxious the moment Maria left, and I couldn't concentrate on a book, couldn't calm myself.

As the sun began to set on the first day, I

called Izzy to me and we sat by the stove —
it was too cold now to sit outdoors come
evening. I brewed myself a cup of tea. Izzy
rested his head on one of my boots and
closed his eyes; I closed mine.

I was already by then in the shadows, I
think, and probably wouldn't be able to
enjoy camping until I'd done enough work to
feel healthier, more myself. When I was able
to love camping again, it would mean that I
was better, stronger.

The next day, Maria came to help bring
me out. We had become close friends by
then, the kind who don't need to be told
what's going on. She gave me a hug, unusual
for this gentle but decidedly undemonstra-
tive person.

"What's that hug for?" I asked, very glad to
see her.

"For the look on your face," she said.

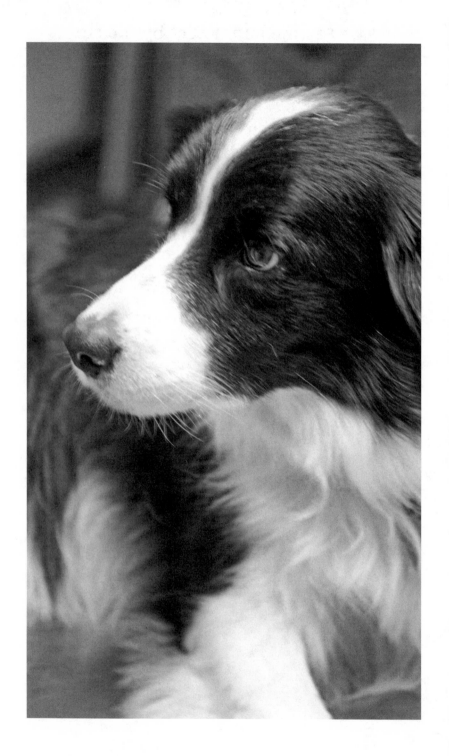

CHAPTER EIGHT: HARRY

The hospice trainers warned us that every experience would be different, that no matter how carefully we prepared, we should expect the unexpected. And it proved to be so.

Harry, a community college professor, had suffered for years with congestive heart failure. He'd had an only partially successful heart transplant in New York City and endured a number of other surgeries, until finally he and his wife had had enough and called hospice. He was spending his final months in the sunroom of their renovated Adirondack-style cabin in nearby Shushan.

Harry and Edra had owned their small hobby farm for several years. He loved animals but especially dogs, border collies in particular; at one time, he'd had a couple of his own, working with a small flock of sheep. He and his dogs went to herding seminars and trials. So the hospice staff thought him a natural for an Izzy visit.

I was told Harry was weak and tired these days, but "fully oriented" and communicative. That made him different from some of the patients we'd been seeing, but what really made Harry unusual was his age: fifty-nine.

Visiting an eighty-year-old dying in a nursing home is one thing; going to see a middle-aged man, someone a year younger than I, was another.

It might be easier to face the end, I thought, if your life had taken its full anticipated course, harder if you were in the midst of things still and conscious that your death was approaching. The social worker warned that Harry was feeling depressed, that his decision to finally let go had been, understandably, difficult.

I often thought of the old adage when I made hospice calls: We will all fall. The people I saw were no different from me, and each reminded me of where life inevitably goes, and reminded me to do good and live well in the meantime.

Harry was more like me than others, though. It was a situation where Izzy and I would simply have to use our judgment and I would help however I could.

The cabin was warm and woodsy, with Shushan's lovely hills and fields stretching outside its big window. We found Harry sitting on a plaid sofa, an iPod tucked into his bathrobe pocket, the TV remote next to him, his computer on a desk behind him.

This was someone very much in my world, not immobilized, demented, or semicomatose. He had more hair than I did, brown flecked with gray, and in addition to his pajamas and robe he was wearing a pair of Nikes.

Yet he was slouched over, his skin pale and his face drained. An oxygen tank stood next to the sofa.

The room around him was filled with books, magazines, and Boston sports paraphernalia — a Red Sox cap, a huge Patriots pennant on the wall. Izzy, like me, appeared a bit taken aback. There was no hospital bed or wheelchair, not much medical equipment at all. Hospice patients experiencing pain are usually medicated, and therefore drowsy, but Harry was perfectly alert. Perhaps he wasn't in pain.

He smiled, perhaps reading our faces. "Expecting worse, were you? I'm glad it doesn't look that bad. Not yet.

"I can get up and walk around," he added, "but not that often. I try to make the trips count."

Izzy, responding to Harry's voice, walked

over and rested his head on Harry's knee, his signature greeting.

"So you're the famous Izzy all the hospice people are talking about," Harry said. "Pleased to meet you. I'm glad you could make time in your busy schedule to see me." After spending time with patients barely able to communicate at all, I was a little startled to encounter someone capable of irony.

Izzy *was* becoming well known, at least in hospice circles. His photo had appeared in a local weekly when we graduated from training, and the nurses and social workers were beginning to talk about him. He was developing a reputation as an intuitive, extremely well-behaved dog who usually managed to find a way to connect, gently and unobtrusively, with patients. Several of those we'd seen had calmed down significantly after Izzy visited, slept more peacefully, and seemed more comfortable being changed, bathed, or medicated. And so we were fielding a growing stream of requests for visits.

If Izzy had a specialty, it was dealing with Alzheimer's and other kinds of dementia. Even when patients were agitated or remote, he seemed able to reach them.

A case like Harry's was, by comparison, much easier. Harry was calm, articulate, fully aware of his surroundings. Izzy didn't have to wait for him to wake up, or deal with outbursts of anger or fear, and certainly not dodge blows. Harry looked very tired, but he remained a gracious host.

And yet, Harry was dying; we wouldn't be there otherwise. The things he was feeling were not obvious to me. But perhaps Izzy could sense them.

As Harry talked to the dog, intermittently asking me a few questions about myself, Izzy clambered up onto the sofa next to him, flopped over, and put his head in Harry's lap. Harry stroked him and seemed moved by his affection. "Why, you *are* a sweetheart, aren't you?"

It occurred to me, watching Izzy and Harry — Edra had gone into a room in the back of the house to do some laundry — that some of Izzy's appeal was that he offered love, unconditionally and purely.

I was glad to be a hospice volunteer, glad to feel helpful, but I couldn't say I loved the patients I saw, or even really came to know them very well. I mostly listened, helped if I could, talked to beleaguered family members if they wanted — and brought Izzy. The patients and family members appreciated my efforts, but they didn't love me, either.

With Izzy it was different. I think he did love them, simply but profoundly, and I think they responded to him in the same way. That was the extraordinary bond I saw him develop with patients, again and again.

I sat, mesmerized, watching Harry light up, have a quiet conversation with Izzy, feel his furry warmth. He appreciated Izzy's absolute and unquestioning devotion; Izzy instinctually appreciated Harry's attention and trust.

Before long, Izzy fell asleep in Harry's lap, and Harry dozed off himself. When Edra came in, carrying a laundry basket — the chores in a hospice home were neverending, I'd found — she was startled to see Izzy and Harry snoozing peacefully on the sofa, Harry's head lolling to one side.

"Wow," she said quietly. "That's beautiful. Beautiful. What a great dog."

We moved to a couch in the adjoining room. Harry had been down, she said, agonizing over his decision to curtail further medical procedures. He was worrying about their two grown children, and also about her. "He feels awfully guilty," she said. "But he is so tired."

She talked, as hospice spouses often did, about their lives together — how they'd met when they were both graduate students at NYU, lived in a half-dozen different places, raised two sons. Harry had always been a fine teacher, patient and dedicated to his students.

During summer breaks they'd traveled widely, she said, and vacationed often in the Adirondacks; thus this cabin-style home. They'd had a great life.

We often encountered this kind of life review in hospice homes, where a spouse, already grieving, was remembering the life they'd shared, almost steeling herself for what came next.

To listen to these stories was an indirect but valuable way in which Izzy and I could help. Izzy's presence gave Harry pleasure, distracted him from his depression, relaxed him to the point of sleep. This, in turn, gave Edra a chance to sit down with me, to think and talk about her husband, perhaps to prepare for his imminent death.

So while Izzy was doing little, he was doing a lot. He was bringing comfort and peace to two people who badly needed it.

We left thirty minutes later, Harry still asleep, Edra beginning to prepare dinner. We'd come back in a few days.

The earliest visits Izzy and I made were usually structured, arranged by hospice officials who often accompanied us to the home to make sure that we got acclimated and that the families were at ease with us.

After that, we could call up and arrange our own visits, as long as we filled out our paperwork.

Generally, I learned, families preferred visits in the morning, when patients tended to have more energy, or in the early afternoon, to break up their long days. But Edra didn't have a preference. We were welcome anytime. She didn't seem to need to be spelled. "I'm happy to have this time with Harry," she said. "I wouldn't miss it."

So Izzy and I visited Harry two or three times a week, usually at mid-afternoon, for an hour or so. Harry liked mysteries, so I brought some along — I liked mysteries myself. I also brought news of Boston sports, which was plentiful online, and CDs of recent Red Sox play-off victories. I wasn't much of a sports fan, but I'd learned enough from Internet stories to talk about Red Sox trade rumors or Bill Belichek's latest outburst.

Izzy became Harry's fast friend, however, without working at it nearly so hard. He'd spring nimbly onto the sofa, where Harry often tucked a biscuit or two between the cushions for Izzy to discover and scarf down. Then Harry rubbed Izzy's belly and talked to him, which Izzy loved even more than treats. He locked in, his eyes wide, staring back at Harry, paying rapt attention.

By the third week, the routine was set: Harry greeted Izzy, plied him with snacks and conversation, talked with me about mystery plots and sports stories I'd printed out from various blogs. He usually fell asleep within forty minutes, Izzy cuddled next to him.

It's not easy to read a dog's behavior, but Izzy was as comfortable here as I'd seen him in any hospice home.

Edra made us some tea and the two of us would talk while Izzy and Harry dozed. We made a good team, Izzy paying more attention to Harry, I to Edra.

Gracious as he was, I thought Harry felt a bit uneasy with human volunteers. Some hospice patients — especially older ones — are lonely, thrilled to have someone to talk to, a new face or a break in routine. Harry, I suspected, didn't really like taking help from people.

Izzy, on the other hand, raised no such issues, posed no emotional conflicts. He was pleased to snuggle alongside him, providing nothing but comfort and affection, requiring nothing but pats. He was a dog.

Izzy, Edra told me, took her husband "off the clock." He seemed to forget about things, to just relax. "It's a gift to him," she said. "And to me."

He took to calling Izzy "the Izster," even suggested I change his name. He asked me about Izzy's past many times, and never tired of hearing our saga. He hadn't forgotten it, I don't think, though his energy was flagging; he simply liked hearing the story.

"Izzy has a good soul," he said. "I never get the impression that he's doing something because he's trained to do it, or because he wants a biscuit. I always get the feeling he likes coming here; he wants to spend time with me." I told him I couldn't really say, but it seemed that way to me as well.

We visited Harry perhaps a dozen times, and then, about the fourth week, I got the call that you should always expect to get but is somehow always surprising: Harry had died peacefully at home the day before, with Edra and the children. I was invited to the funeral home in Queensbury for the memorial service. Izzy, too.

Among the photos arranged on an easel in the chapel was one of Harry and Izzy napping together on the sofa, which I'd taken and given to Edra.

After the psalms and hymns, Izzy, wearing his hospice photo ID, sat next to Edra and greeted a long line of mourners. Everyone seemed to know who he was, and many people, stooping to give him a scratch or a pat, thanked him for the time he spent with Harry.

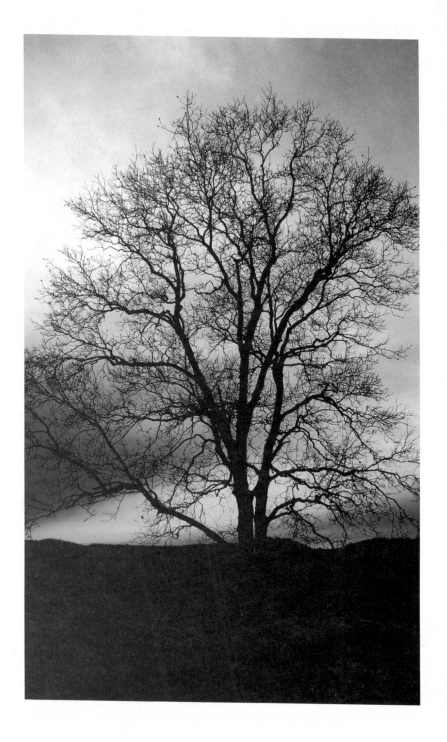

CHAPTER NINE:
INTO THE SHADOWS

Depression: 1. severe despondency and dejection, especially when long-lasting and accompanied by physical symptoms. 2. a sunken place or hollow.
— *Oxford English Dictionary*

Of the two, I liked the second definition better.

I don't really know exactly when I found myself in a sunken place. My attempts to ward off the bad feelings, to right myself, didn't seem to be having much effect.

Perhaps I knew I was sunk that morning when I came out the back door toting the trash and Lulu, my favorite donkey, began her joyous bray. It was an odd, breathy sound that usually lifted my spirits, but that day I felt too worn down to bring her the cookie she expected, and I thought her braying turned from a greeting to a reproach. I love Lulu, and I've been delighted to bring her a cookie every morning. I wonder if she knew before I did that it would be weeks before I would bring her the next one.

Another day, Annie popped in to ask if I was ready to move some large round bales of hay into the pasture for Elvis and the crew, a task that involved my tractor. No, I wasn't ready. Could she and her husband Joe handle it? I wondered.

Annie was agreeable as always, but also clearly startled. Normally there's nothing I love more than firing up the big orange Kubota, sticking an Aretha Franklin disc into its CD player, and spearing a round bale or two for Elvis and Harold and Luna. But I didn't feel up for it. In fact, I didn't climb into the tractor for nearly two months. Instead, I went upstairs for a nap that day and listened to Joe maneuver my tractor out to the pasture. I didn't even sleep.

This trough had started slowly, indirectly. Trouble sleeping. Fatigue. Dejection, anxiety, an inability to take pleasure in things that usually cheered me. A loss of energy. Unwanted memories and dreams from childhood, a dark time I had no desire to revisit. I had struggled with depression when I was young, but not in a long, long time.

In some ways, this bout ought not have

been surprising. I'd been through a long, difficult ordeal with friends struggling with a number of issues, and I'd put much of my own life aside to try to help them through. I'd also finished an extended and challenging book tour, dealt with the difficulties of diabetes. Something in these experiences had opened up some old, deep veins of sorrow.

My move to the farm had been enormously exhilarating, I reflected. But it was also more difficult, more physically and emotionally demanding than many people — who fantasize about a bucolic life, surrounded by animals — might realize. It had been a wonderful time, but also costly, and draining.

And isolating, in some ways. Paula and Emma, both committed New Yorkers, loved to spend time with me on the farm, but weren't here much of the time. Paula was busy teaching her fall semester at Columbia, and Emma was immersed in writing a book. They seemed busy to me, distracted; perhaps I was imagining it, but our conversations struck me as hurried, superficial, leaving me feeling cut off. And November can be a bleak month upstate — dark, cold, rainy, and gloomy.

Apart from them, I was no longer in touch

with anyone from my former life, not from our twenty-plus years in New Jersey or from the media world, not from my own family. My parents were dead; I hadn't spoken to my brother in years, or to other relatives; I had only occasional contact with my sister. I'd made some wonderful friends upstate, but my work and other demands had pulled me away from them, too, left me struggling to keep up with them, to pay attention.

As much as I loved the place, my move upstate had been disconnecting. I'd uprooted myself from a world I'd known for a long time, to a new life in a place where I could never totally belong.

I stopped by the Bedlam Corners variety store for a half-gallon of milk one day just before Thanksgiving. "That dog guy on the hill is fixing up another barn," one guy in fatigues was saying to another.

"Yeah, must be nice to have money," said the other.

It was jarring to realize they were talking about me — the refugee, the outsider.

So, not surprisingly perhaps, I felt plunged into a long retreat inward and backward, deep into my own psyche, into fears and anxieties and loss. At first, I was in what the twelve-step people like to call a state of denial: I didn't fully recognize these problems or their symptoms, or understand how helpless and confused I'd become.

The shadows crept up on me until, suddenly, I was enveloped.

The animals, usually animated and eager around me, began to seem a bit sluggish. Dogs are extraordinarily sensitive to humans' moods; when I'm up, they're excited, too, ready to go. When I'm not, they become slower, flatter, less energetic.

Just as Izzy reflects the feelings of the hospice patients he visits, my dogs reflect me and what I'm feeling at the moment. They can't know what I'm thinking, but they instinctively read my moods. It is, perhaps, why our relationships with them can be so meaningful.

I got that something was off, but not what. After I confided to Elvis that I was in a funk, I simply soldiered on with my life, a mistake, and a costly one.

I wasn't prepared for the physical symptoms of depression — a sense of moving slowly, of utter exhaustion. It was difficult to talk to Paula or Emma, or to my friends. It was hard to get up in the morning, walk the dogs, crank myself up for work.

Sitting at my desk, I felt distracted, reaching for a cup of coffee, then stopping mid-reach as a stray thought interrupted. I called

Paula, then quickly wanted to get off the phone.

Meals became perfunctory, tossing something — anything — into the microwave. I drank a glass of milk, made some tea. My blood glucose numbers jumped too high, and when I called my doctor, the nurse asked if I was experiencing any stress or emotional problems. I said I supposed I was. Well, she said, that probably explained it.

At night, which comes early and totally during upstate winters, I kept looking at my watch, hoping it was time to go to bed. I couldn't stay awake long enough to read; then I couldn't fall asleep. I forgot to brush my teeth, shave, do the laundry. My woodland walks with the dogs, a happy routine that anchored the day for me, became shorter, obligatory.

The one party I was certain sensed something was up was the ever-vigilant Rose, who misses nothing and feels responsible for everything.

Rose is all instinct, all work. Monitoring the farm and its environs are her terrain, her task. If a ewe wanders too near an electrical fence, Rose knows it. If I drop my cell phone in the pasture, Rose will go to it first thing next morning. She's constantly taking inventory, noticing what's new, different, aberrant. I may never have a stronger bond with any nonhuman creature than with this dog, who moved with me to the farm when she was just six months old and has been by my side ever since.

Now she stayed unusually close, slept by my feet, hopped up onto the bed at night — a rare thing — and watched me. Normally, she maintained her own space, going from window to window, checking on the sheep. Suddenly, her focus had shifted; she was lying next to me at the computer and on the couch.

I'm Rose's connection to sheep; if something happens to me, she will not get to herd, and that's important to her. Possibly that was her rationale. At any rate, I had become her work, and she took her work seriously. Every time I looked up, Rose was watching me intently. Something was different, and she knew it and was on the alert.

One morning, I left the other dogs in the fenced yard and took Rose out for a walk alone. She normally races far ahead of me on the path through the woods, circling back when I call. This time she stayed by my side, sniffing here and there, but hanging close.

"You know something, don't you, girl?" I said, confident that she did. She looked at me curiously, filing notes away for future reference.

I was feeling as murky physically as I was emotionally. Vaguely nauseous and dizzy, I had headaches; often, I felt sore. I grew sluggish, disoriented.

I love to go out to dinner, a respite from the dark cold days of winter. I stopped. I love going to movies — anyplace, anytime, by myself. But not then.

I had stopped visiting Elvis, stopped herding sheep and visiting the barn cats in their recesses. Parts of me were shutting down.

I actually frightened myself. It's not possible to live this way, not a life as I've known it.

And I was depressed about being depressed, and embarrassed. I didn't want to tell anyone what I was going through, didn't want to be pitied or fussed over, another focus of people's anxiety in an already anxious world. In my mind, I was a helper, in control, filled with answers, not a victim who'd lost control and suddenly had none.

Yet I wrote every day, good stuff and bad, with heavy hands and a disconnected head. I think I was afraid of what might happen if I stopped, so I wrote and wrote and wrote.

■ ■ ■ ■

Trying to fight back, I ordered boxes of books, more Thomas Merton, C. S. Lewis, more Joseph Campbell, St. Augustine — plus guides to digital photography — and sat up late poring over them, trying to learn what better minds than mine had to teach about loss and sadness.

Meanwhile, I tried to reestablish my routines. I got up at dawn to walk the dogs with Annie, a cheerful person whose visits meant a lot to me; she is a person of habit, of solidity. It would have made her uncomfortable to know that I waited eagerly for her to come through the door, hoping she would walk with me, even though normally I cherished my walks with the dogs alone.

Photography helped, too. I took my camera with me everywhere. I took pictures in the woods, in the barns. I took so many photos of the dogs that they probably thought the camera permanently attached to my hands. I began to see the world in a different light, literally; to think visually, to keep a tripod in my Blazer, just in case. I drove around for miles, stopping at collapsing barns, glowing diners, car dealerships, dairy farms.

And I turned to the people I cared about.

I had, piece by piece, come to feel disconnected from my family, my farm, my animals, and my friends. But it probably saved my hide to realize, eventually, that none of these had become disconnected from me. That told me, once I could hear it, that I would be all right.

I called my friend Becky, the most religiously devout person I knew, and sucked up her faith like a sponge. Sometimes we met for dinner at the Barn and sat in front of the vast stone fireplace talking about grief and loss. Becky had lost her husband, Bill, to colon cancer nine years earlier, and she told me about the stages of grief, and about the faith that propelled her forward and gave her ground to stand on.

"You will be okay," she announced one night. "You are strong and you will figure things out." I felt weak, but I also felt that I would figure things out. Was there much choice?

I visited my friend Maria in her artist's studio, and she told me night after night that I was resilient, I would recover and be fine.

"How do you know I'll be fine?" I asked.

"I don't know how," she said. "I just know."

Sometimes, I believed her. We sat in front of the woodstove in her studio, drinking tea and eating the popcorn that I brought over, and I remember thinking that people who have friends like this and can talk to them on windswept and spooky nights can survive.

Some mornings, Maria would come help me out with the animals. She seemed to know, like Rose, when to appear and when to stay away. A lot of attention, too much scrutiny, would have done me in, I think.

My poet friend Mary Kellogg called almost daily to ask how I was. "You're a good man," she kept telling me. I trusted Mary; if she said that, it might be true.

Paula came up to keep me company, but she also struggled to communicate with me. A rational person, the experience of mental illness was alien to her, and very disturbing. She cared, she sympathized, but she despaired of knowing how to help. "If anyone else you knew was going through this, anyone at all, you would tell them to get a shrink," she said pointedly.

Heeding her fears, and knowing there was a limit to what even a loving family and friends could do, I did locate a therapist in Saratoga.

Meanwhile, Izzy and I held faithfully to our hospice work, which, oddly, was not depressing or discouraging at all, but uplifting, not something that drained me but that replenished me. The very thing most people warned me against was helping to pull me through. Hospice work with my sweet dog allowed me to still feel good about myself, and it provided badly needed perspective.

Here the work was clear, the boundaries chillingly defined. We were needed. We did good. We helped. How strange that visits to the dying cheered me more than almost anything else.

It's not only a cliché, I thought: Everything *is* a gift in its own bizarre way. Depression was bringing me a stream of presents. Paula made it clear how much she loved and supported me. So did my daughter, Emma. I was reconnecting with friends. I was taking some good pictures. I was writing with new insight. I was beginning to be honest with myself.

I had reached a black and unhealthy state of mind and, to be frank, I was terrified I wouldn't get out no matter how people tried to reassure me. Nothing mattered much but waiting for the ordeal to end. The "gifts," though welcome, did not make up for the bleakness, or quell my fear that I'd lost the ability to live and survive in the world.

"This will be a painful time for you," my new shrink told me the first time we met.

"We have a lot of things to figure out."
Hurry up, I thought. I'm sixty.

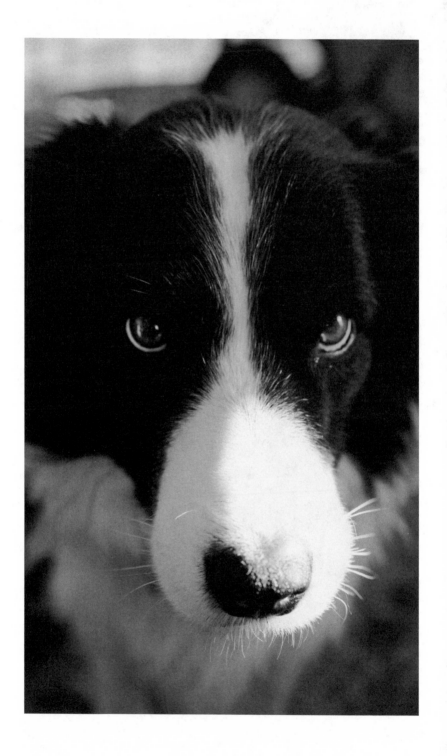

CHAPTER TEN:
TIMMY

When Izzy and I arrived at Timmy's house, just north of Argyle, a private-duty nurse was on her way down the walk. This development of modest, newish homes stretched across what must have been farmland once. Dairy farms still surrounded the new houses on three sides, fragrant with silage and manure.

The nurse introduced herself to me — Rae was her name — and headed for the driveway. Then she paused and actually walked back toward us.

"I've been doing this for quite a while," she said. "But this one is a bit rough. Just get set."

I appreciated the caution. Some deaths, I'd learned, seemed natural, accepted, even welcome sometimes. Some didn't. Inside this split-level, a seven-year-old boy was dying of a brain tumor. He lived with his mother, Marla, who had called hospice care just a few weeks earlier.

She'd been on family leave from the state transportation department, where she worked as an auditor, for two months, ever since Timmy had left the hospital in Albany. Keith, the hospice volunteer coordinator, cautioned that Marla had been sitting with her gravely ill son for many weeks and was, understandably, struggling.

Now, I was told, the boy was close to death, heavily medicated, fading in and out of consciousness.

This was different from helping an elderly woman with Alzheimer's die comfortably. Different for me, and different, I imagined, for Izzy.

A slim young woman with dark hair and deep circles beneath her eyes answered the doorbell, glanced at our hospice tags, and asked us in. She was genial and welcoming, but she looked depleted, utterly exhausted. We sat with her at the dining room table. "Timmy loves dogs," she told us. "He still misses Ginger, the golden retriever we used to have. She got hit by a car last spring and we had to put her down, about the same time Timmy got sick." Marla leaned over and rubbed Izzy's head.

A Disney video was playing softly in the background. This was becoming familiar:

The families of the dying don't want them to feel alone, not for a minute, so there's almost always music or a TV on, voices in the background.

I noticed, too, the medicinal smell in the small, neat house, a mix of ointments and salves and antiseptics.

Izzy surveyed the room, his gaze lighting on the hospital bed set up in the middle of the living room. Also increasingly familiar: living rooms serving as convenient places for sick people, a space where they can be comforted and monitored by family, friends, doctors, nurses, and social workers. It keeps them in the middle of activity, not shut away, and provides easy access to kitchens and TVs.

In the bed, his head swathed in bandages, an IV dripping into his left arm, a boy lay watching us curiously, his head resting on a pillow, his face and forehead swollen and disfigured from surgical efforts to reduce pain and swelling. The lines of his thin body were visible under the sheets and blankets. He was a beautiful child, dark-eyed with wavy brown hair peeking out from beneath the bandages. A table near the bed was layered with stuffed animals and electronic toys, books and puzzles, and lots of get-well cards.

Marla went over to Timmy to straighten his blankets, check on the IV, stroke his cheek. I looked down at Izzy, who had locked in on the boy in the bed.

"Timmy," I heard Marla say, "there's a dog named Izzy who has come to visit with you."

Timmy looked back at us and smiled. We were welcome. I took a deep breath, collected myself, and tried to remember what we'd been taught. In normal life, people outside of emergency rooms and intensive care units don't often get to meet dying boys.

There's a loneliness to dying, though it's not necessarily the sort of loneliness I might have expected. People who are dying often seemed reconciled to it, accepting, gathering themselves for the process. Their loneliness, it seemed to me, came more from the fact that the rest of the world cringed, shied away, backed off. Often families we saw were alone with the experience because the rest of us simply couldn't or didn't know how to cope with it.

This, I think, was one reason Izzy meant so much to people: He bothered to come.

"This is unbearable, so I understand why nobody comes by," Marla said. I thought she'd read my thoughts. "His grandmother can't do it anymore. She's got a heart condition and when she comes, she just bursts into tears. Once she fainted, and that was upsetting for Timmy. Poor thing, her doctor told her not to visit anymore.

"When Timmy first got sick, his teacher came by with the class, but it was too hard for the kids, and some of their parents wouldn't even let them come along. Not one of them has come back." People couldn't stand the idea of a child dying. Even Timmy's father, who lived a couple of hours away, was down to twice-weekly visits.

"He said he felt helpless," she told me. "Like there isn't anything he could do. Well, there's a lot he could do. But I'm not going to ask, if he doesn't know himself." She allowed herself a short, sad laugh.

"I can't blame anyone," Marla sighed. "I can hardly bear to be here myself. Though of course I wouldn't be anywhere else, no matter what. But we manage, we manage . . . We do the best we can."

Still, the isolation must have been painful. I recognized Marla's sense of being shunned. She was intensely grateful for the visits from hospice workers. She was also going online, where she'd found a website for mothers in this awful circumstance. The priest from their church came by regularly — "And you know what? Sara, who works with me at the DOT, she comes by once a week with food, videos, spends some time with me. I love her visits, and the food's a big help. I eat it all week, and don't have to cook. Timmy doesn't eat much anymore, mostly just those protein shakes in cans."

She made another turn through the living room, plumping Timmy's pillow, adjusting the volume on the video, trying to get her son to take a swallow of something from a teaspoon — then returned to me, looking worn and sad. She was losing altitude; you could see her droop.

"I've done everything I can think of, but he's still suffering," she said to me, her voice catching. "I wish I could do more. I should be."

Izzy, meanwhile, had walked slowly over to the side of Timmy's bed and sat staring at the boy. His demeanor was businesslike, professional, as if to say: If these two people are going to be over there, talking, I'll come check things out over here and get to work. Timmy turned his head; I thought he saw Izzy, but I couldn't tell.

Marla continued; I didn't dare to interrupt. Hospice nurses, volunteers, and social workers had been visiting the home regularly for weeks and everyone was touched and moved by how dutiful she was, how loving and attentive. Just watching her drift back and forth to Timmy, checking his bandages, kissing him on the nose, taking his temperature, looking into his eyes, whispering soothingly into his ear, I couldn't see how she could possibly be doing more.

We had role-played for this during training. I'd heard nearly the same words from my partner in that exercise, which now seemed to have happened long ago — this notion of not trying hard enough, not being able to turn back death with sheer will and love and courage, as in some heartwarming movie. I'd heard it often since.

I remembered the lesson: You're not there to cheer people up or deny the reality of their lives. Meet Marla where she is, let her have her grief and loss. Don't try to take them from her, or diminish them by suggesting she should just decide to feel better. Sitting with her, it was clear that she couldn't, and might not for a very long time.

So I didn't say what I was thinking, what I would normally have said: Marla, you're wrong. You're doing everything, more than almost anyone could. You are a great mother, and a loving person. Don't beat yourself up.

Instead I listened, and after a few minutes I asked, "Marla, do you think Timmy might like to meet Izzy now?"

She walked me toward the bed, where

Timmy lay, his eyes closed at the moment, then open again. Izzy came around with me to the far side of the bed.

I flipped my hand, the "up" command, and Izzy hopped lightly onto the foot of the bed. He used his signature method, lying down and then moving slowly toward his patient. In a moment he rested his head on Timmy's shoulder, and Timmy turned to look at Izzy and broke into a smile wide enough that I could see a missing tooth.

"Hey," the boy whispered. "What?" He looked a little disoriented, surprised but pleased, as if he thought he were dreaming. I guess he was trying to figure out the sudden appearance of this attentive animal by his side. "Are you my new dog?"

"Sort of," I said, introducing Izzy and myself. "He's going to be your part-time dog for a while, Timmy. He's going to live on my farm but come here and visit you when you need to see him."

"I can't keep him?" he asked. "He can't stay here?"

No, I said, Izzy had a home, and he was loved there. But he'd come by pretty often, and they could spend time together. That way, I added, you don't have to walk or feed him. It seemed a good deal to Timmy; at least, he didn't question it further. He moved his small hand to ruffle Izzy's fur.

That was all Izzy needed. He wriggled around, avoiding the plastic IV line, and put his head on Timmy's chest.

"Hey," he said to his mother, in a soft, slightly halting voice. "Izzy is awesome." This was, I could see, an instant friendship.

Timmy asked a few questions about Izzy — where he came from, who had named him (not me), did I have any other animals on the farm.

He was bright, cheerful, polite. Marla murmured that he hadn't been talking much in the past week or so, so Izzy had made an impression, gotten Timmy interested. Izzy lay on the bed for perhaps fifteen minutes, then carefully hopped off and sat on the floor.

I couldn't really tell why. He'd developed his own way of working with hospice patients. He had his own clock, his own sense of when to approach and when not to, when to lie on the bed and cuddle, when to take a break and go curl up in a corner. In this case, Izzy's next stop was Marla; he put his head in her hand. She stroked him absently for a minute or two, and then he found a space under a chair and went to sleep.

Timmy was asleep, too, his eyes closed, his breathing soft and rhythmic.

Marla and I sat down again in the dining

alcove. She brought me a glass of water and resumed talking. I listened, nodded, wondered how she got through any given day.

Timmy was such a normal second-grader, she said. He loved using her computer, playing video games, riding his bike when she shooed him out of the house. He didn't have a lot of friends, just two or three kids from the neighborhood. But that was enough. He was a happy, presumably healthy boy.

"He started getting headaches, a swelling around the eyes a few months ago," she said. Their regular pediatrician looked so upset examining Timmy that she knew instantly that something was seriously wrong.

"I guess the really hard thing, especially since he came home, since he's under hospice care, is the time," she continued. "I had no idea how long a day could be. And I start thinking, 'If there is a God, *Wake up. Stop this. Deal with this.*' I love him so much. It's lonely, and it's so sad." She stopped herself then, with an almost visible effort. "How great for you to come here with Izzy. He really cheered Timmy up."

We went back over to say whispered goodbyes to Timmy. "I think we'll be back," I told Izzy as we left.

We were back two days later. I called the hospice office and said we'd be available to come by as often as needed. I thought Izzy had even cheered Marla up a bit, in addition to Timmy. He'd even paused to cuddle with a surprised and delighted hospice aide who was coming in as we were leaving.

Our visits took on a pattern. Timmy was weak and medicated and couldn't stay awake long. What he liked was for Izzy to snuggle next to him, so he could put his hand on Izzy's head or shoulder and then go to sleep, as if with a large stuffed animal. We let Izzy and Timmy lie together that way while I sat on the sofa nearby with Marla, who talked about what the last couple of days had been like: small triumphs (Timmy had eaten a little pudding) and losses (he couldn't really play video games anymore). She also repeated her belief that she wasn't helping him enough, that she wished she could do more.

Timmy seemed to be sleeping more often and more deeply as our visits continued, and speaking less. But he was clearly aware of Izzy, smiling when we came in, and then talking to him a bit while they settled in for their nap together. I couldn't tell what Timmy was saying, but Marla and I agreed that their conversations ought to be private.

It was hard to look over and see this beautiful but wrenching sight, Izzy and Timmy lying next to one another, Timmy holding

Izzy, clutching him sometimes, talking and sleeping, then talking and sleeping some more.

We came several times a week for a few weeks. I brought Marla some books and CDs, and we talked — or rather I listened while she talked — about Timmy, how much she loved him, how she hated to see him suffer, how she knew he wasn't going to make it, and how she would probably never get over it.

I did veer from my training a bit one afternoon, because I could hardly bear her berating herself — I had even reported this to the hospice social worker, who was already well aware of it. "Marla," I said, sipping the tea she had made me while Izzy and Timmy slept on the bed, "I hope you will come to see one day that this isn't your fault. I'm sure you will." Then I stopped myself from going further and listened.

Timmy had grown quieter recently. Apart from murmuring to Izzy, he didn't say much, at least not to me. But Marla thought the dog helped him sleep better, to feel more comfortable.

I had brought him two pictures of Izzy, and both were taped up on the wall alongside his bed. I had a stuffed border collie I brought on book tours, and I named it "Izzy" and

gave it to Timmy, who kept it next to his pillow.

Izzy had a routine now. He'd figured things
out like an office worker who'd been com-
muting for years on the same train. He came
in, greeted Marla, looked at me for the okay,
then hopped onto the bed to lie with Timmy.
The communication between the two had
become wordless. Timmy no longer said
much to Izzy, Izzy no longer looked for any
verbal cues from me. They just held one another, an embrace that rendered speech unnecessary.

After a while, Izzy no longer bothered to
look at me or even to greet Marla until later.
He went quickly and directly to Timmy, as if
he sensed the urgency, the passing days and
the limits on their time together. When we
pulled up to Timmy's house, he almost raced
to get to the door and inside.

Then, one day, as happens in hospice, we
came to the door, and Marla was there with
several other people, all crying. I understood.

This was the thing I had the most trouble
with in hospice work. I could handle the
sickness, deal with the grief and the death.
The hardest part was to show up at the
home of someone whose lives Izzy and I had
entered so intimately, and to find them sim-

ply gone. Hospice volunteers were not generally the people called when someone died; family members and friends were far more important. So sometimes we didn't know that our job was over until we showed up and someone was just not there.

I took a deep breath when I saw Marla, and she fell into my arms. "Oh, Jon, Izzy," she said, weeping. "Timmy passed this morning, and it was so peaceful, I was glad for that. I am so grateful to Izzy." She knelt and wrapped her arms around him.

Then Marla stood up, and Izzy went into the living room, looking around, darting from one spot to another, surrounded by a roomful of strangers. I pointed to Timmy's bed, and Izzy hopped up on it, and lay still.

I could explain little of what had passed between that poor boy and my dog, but this I did understand: Izzy was saying good-bye.

CHAPTER ELEVEN: PAUL

On paper, this patient, Paul, sounded commonplace. Izzy and I had encountered his condition half a dozen times, more frequently than any other — an Alzheimer's patient in steep decline. When his wife, Danielle, met us at the door, I saw the expression I'd come to know: grief tinged with exhaustion.

The house was a small bungalow, perhaps a converted barn; judging from the paint and trim and slate roof, it had probably been a costly renovation. From the door, I could see Paul, seated in a high-backed chair in the center of the room, close to the television.

Danielle was happy to see Izzy and me. There had been few visitors lately, she said, almost all from hospice. Next week their children would be flying in from Seattle for a few days, and that would be welcome. But today, she said quietly, taking my coat, was a lonely day.

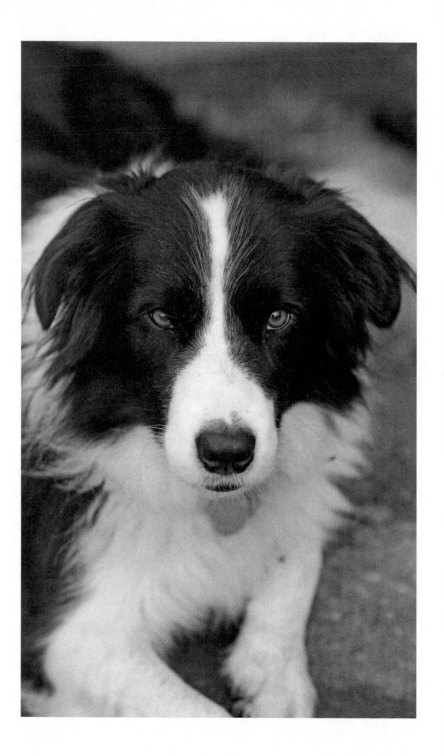

Danielle seemed a gentle person, soft-spoken. Offering me a seat on the sofa and a cup of tea, she told me a bit about Paul, about his fiery career as a prosecutor with the state attorney general's office, and how much she'd relished the peaceful decade they'd had here in the countryside since he left Albany. Politics, she said, was a tough business, and so was law enforcement.

They'd enjoyed their retirement. Paul was a hunter and fisherman. They drove down to Florida's west coast for the winters, where Paul fantasized about buying and operating a charter fishing boat.

Healthy spouses seemed to need to talk about their marriages this way, how they'd begun and evolved and survived. Before long, I'd know where they'd met, where they'd lived, when the kids were born, where they used to vacation. What kind of a man he was, how glad she was to be caring for him now, how difficult it was to see him like this. I had the sense that they were collecting all the good memories, years of love and affection, unconsciously preparing for the time when they'd have only those memories to rely on.

I was always amazed at how uncomplaining these spouses were — wives, mostly — accepting death but determined to be faithful, making sure their loved ones were well cared for to the end. I rarely saw anybody take a shortcut, forget a medication, put off bathing or changing, react angrily to the unconscious provocations of the terminally ill. Once strong and competent and articulate men were much reduced; they couldn't control their bodily functions or their language any longer and sometimes lashed out fiercely at the people they most loved. Yet from somewhere these women summoned extraordinary reservoirs of love, patience, and commitment.

"He's been so agitated lately," Danielle said. "Last night when I got him into bed he threw the pillow at me, and I said, 'Paul, I know you hate being in this position, and I love you.'" She started to tear up. I said nothing; there was nothing to say.

As I listened to Danielle, I saw that Paul was asleep in his big chair, his head supported on a pillow affixed to a headstand, a bit like a barber's chair. I hadn't seen one of those before.

Next to him, on a hospital bed, sat a pile of books — mysteries, I saw, and some topical nonfiction. Danielle read to him, I supposed. From the hospice report, it seemed unlikely that Paul could read any longer, or communicate much at all.

Danielle was clearly working hard. The room, tastefully and expensively furnished, was spotless, with fresh flowers on almost every surface. There wasn't a trace of medicinal or other odors, though I could see that Paul was wearing incontinence briefs.

Smells had been a concern of mine and of the hospice people, because dogs have such sensitive noses. I wasn't sure how Izzy would react to someone in diapers. But he never seemed to notice, or react in any way that I could see.

Paul had been restless lately, Danielle said, struggling to avoid his medication, resisting her touch. Though he'd loved dogs, and hunted with them, she wasn't sure how he'd respond now, in this state. But Izzy was by now quite experienced at dealing with this condition. He would wait, back off if necessary, then approach slowly.

When it was time to meet Paul, Izzy and I moved around the couch to Paul's chair. I could see him more clearly now: tall, lean to the point of gauntness, still handsome, with lots of shaggy white hair. He wore a flannel shirt and sweatpants, with oddly spotless white running shoes. Of course they were immaculate, I realized; they hadn't been worn outside the house.

"Paul hasn't spoken coherently in two

years," Danielle said quietly. "That's hard, because I used to go see him in court, and boy, he was something."

I wished I could also have heard Paul addressing juries; even now, you could see the man's presence, his stature.

Izzy approached in his understated way, sliding his head under Paul's hand. Paul blinked awake. Suddenly, feeling Izzy's ears, he said, quite clearly, "Good dog!"

Danielle, excited, walked over.

"Paul," she said. "Paul. This is Izzy, a dog from hospice. Izzy is here with Jon, a volunteer. They've come to see you."

Paul ignored Danielle, or perhaps didn't hear her. He was staring at Izzy, repeating the same phrase over and over, in different ways and with different inflections: "*Good dog. Good. Good dog. Good dog.*"

Izzy tilted his head the way dogs do when they're curious or puzzled, but he sat still, locked in, apparently satisfied with the response.

When we left, a few minutes later, Danielle asked us to please come again. To hear her once-eloquent husband form words — even just two words — was a wonder.

Two days later, therefore, we were back. Paul was wide awake, this time wearing a cardigan sweater; he'd had a haircut and smelled of fresh cologne. He sat in his modified chair, turned toward the door, and when Izzy and I came in, Paul broke into a wide grin. I felt sure that, before he became ill, he had a strong handshake.

Izzy, wasting no time with preliminaries, trotted over and put his head on Paul's lap. Paul exclaimed "Good dog!" again, several times; he practically beamed.

"He always loved dogs — and kids," Danielle said, bringing me tea. "He always stopped to say hello whenever we met a dog. This is definitely touching something in him. He's been in that chair for almost two years and never looked so happy."

Paul had been markedly less agitated, too, she thought; after our first visit, he'd slept well and long at night. I knew the significance of that, why she sounded so appreciative: When hospice patients sleep well, so do the people taking care of them. Danielle looked better than she had on our first visit, more rested.

I helped Danielle wash dishes in the kitchen while Izzy maneuvered onto the chair next to Paul and Paul stroked his head. She had some phone calls to return, so she went into the study and I sat on the sofa across from Paul and watched him with my dog, Paul's hand on Izzy's slender nose.

They were both asleep.

It was one of the few times since I'd been volunteering that I had nothing to do, nobody to listen to; I found it curiously peaceful.

I took a sip of the tea Danielle had made and watched Izzy, his chest rising and falling rhythmically. Paul looked at ease, too.

I had time to mull a bit about what I was doing here, how we'd come to this point. I was at one of those stages of life where, as Joseph Campbell put it, the mask you are wearing cracks and you fall inward, into your own psyche.

I'd thought I was at the apogee, the pinnacle of my life, but now I saw that I wasn't really, that I'd lost some of my power and strength, and was perhaps fighting to do more than was possible, to handle more than was reasonable, to keep the center intact. I'd lost my bearings about who I really was and where I was, and was neglecting old issues by bulling ahead on the strength of my own punishing personality.

On the farm, I'd come to see that my animals managed to avoid, almost entirely by instinct, the dramas that humans create for themselves. I envied them.

In this room, with this vital and beloved man ready to pass from this life, I particularly envied Izzy his clarity. He knew what he was here for; his instincts told him what to do. This confidence, competence, and innate affection were what people at the end of their lives appreciated in Izzy, his simple, clear sense of himself and his purpose.

Doing hospice work together had changed me, although I doubted it had changed Izzy. When you see people leaving the world, you can't help reflecting, considering your own place there.

It's disconcerting to lose track of where you are in life, but hospice work will remind you quickly to take stock and be aware. Soon enough, hospice dogs and their befuddled masters will be paying you a call.

We visited Paul several times a week for perhaps a month. I enjoyed coming to this house. Danielle was loving and gracious, doting on her husband; Paul's buoyant good nature seemed to shine right through his illness. Watching him light up when Izzy came through the door was wonderful.

Even if his vocabulary didn't increase, Paul seemed more animated, more verbal, calmer. Mostly, he and Izzy just sat together, as Paul praised him and ran his hand along his head and back. But I noticed Paul also watching me more, reacting more attentively when I spoke to him, seeming more curious about who I was and what I was doing there. I made a note of this in the volunteer report I filed, that Paul was more alert and responsive during Izzy's visits.

After our ninth or tenth visit, I got a call from the hospice social worker. She wanted me to know that Paul had begun to use other phrases, that his condition was no longer declining, that his health and his orientation had actually improved.

The hospice doctors had therefore decided to take him off their rolls; he was no longer, in their view, declining and close to death. This had happened once or twice before, she said, but it was rare.

She wanted me to know that Danielle and the hospice nurse credited Izzy with this startling turnaround. Paul appeared to be returning, noticeably though probably temporarily, to the world.

"We don't understand it," she said. "But we can all see it. Please thank Izzy for us."

I called for Izzy, told him the good news (he seemed pleased to hear it), and we drove the half hour to Paul's house to say a different sort of good-bye than we'd expected.

Danielle opened the door and threw her arms around me. Paul sat smiling in his special chair. "Hey, good dog!" he said, nodding his head up and down, up and down.

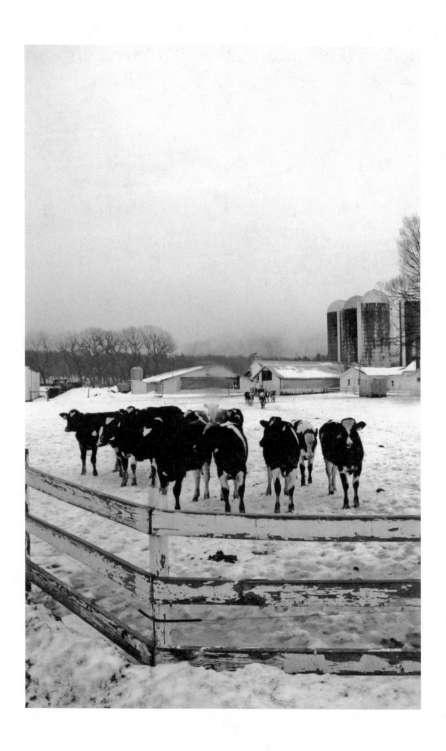

Chapter Twelve: My Big Sister

A few days after one of my camping trips, I woke up in the farmhouse and found I could hardly climb out of bed.

Izzy crept out from underneath the bed, where he slept, Rose was at my feet, and both dogs looked at me curiously. We're almost always up and about at dawn, and it was already light.

Normally, I love mornings on the farm. I walk the dogs through the woods, distribute cookies to donkeys, check the barn for eggs. I trade insults with the goats, give Elvis a smooch on his big nose, then sling my camera over my shoulder and head out in search of something striking to shoot. I wander the place like George Washington surveying his lands.

Not this morning. I felt nearly doubled over, half-paralyzed by a kind of pain that, for once, didn't stem from my hapless back or bad ankle, but from a different place, somewhere around my stomach, heart, throat. Somewhere in my psyche.

I didn't want to take pictures, walk the dogs, or feed the donkeys. Even picking up the phone for my morning check-in with Paula seemed too much. I forced myself to shower and dress.

I tried to write that day; I didn't have much success, didn't like what emerged. I walked the dogs in the woods, barely conscious of their antics and the beauty around us. I felt like a creaky old airplane whose engines were cutting out, one by one; the silence was alarming.

Dusk came early these days, and the nights were terribly cold. I'm rarely lonely on the farm, but this night the loneliness was piercing. For the first time, I was afraid. I couldn't run the farm like this. I couldn't work like this. I couldn't live like this.

As often happens when fears from the past well up, I thought of my sister. Jane is two years older. When we were children, we were profoundly close. Our bedrooms adjoined each other, and we talked one another to sleep every night. We shared the extraordinary bond of traumatized kids. Our parents were both disturbed and angry and our house a fearful place. We experienced things children shouldn't, kept secrets too dark to know.

When Jane was eight, loving and smart and already hurting, she took me down into the basement and told me that our parents hated her, that she wanted to die. She was beginning to break down even then, picked to pieces by people who couldn't grasp how troubled or sensitive she was.

I spent much of my youth trying — and failing, always — to get her help. I went to priests and rabbis and Quaker meetings. I went to the police. I talked to relatives, to kindly neighbors on the block, to charitable groups and counselors. And I battled with my parents day after day, year after year.

Nobody came to help, and my sister's troubles worsened. She broke down in college, locked herself in her bedroom for years, smoked and drank and took drugs. Later on, divorced, she couldn't take care of her two children, who had to be sent elsewhere to live. She was drowning.

For years, we largely lost touch. She lurched from one addiction and obsession to another. She hurt people. She hurt herself. She hurt me.

For a while, I decided that the safety of my new family — Paula and Emma — required me to stay away from the old one, and I did.

I was right, I think.

But I never stopped wondering and worrying about Jane. When she found me, a few years ago, I was amazed to learn that she was sharing a life with animals and considering a move from Massachusetts to upstate New York. She had gotten herself help and was stronger, though still on the fragile side. She rescued dogs — Newfoundlands with heart disease, mostly. She was hoping to move her ailing menagerie to the country, and add to it — goats, chickens, maybe even a donkey.

Thereafter, we talked on the phone from time to time. She mostly asked about my dogs, and I asked about hers; that was safe ground. Then, a year after I moved to my farm, she moved to hers, and we talked about barns and vets and woodstoves. She told me, in one wintertime conversation, that there were some feral sheep living — and starving — in the woods nearby, and she wondered if Rose, whom I had bragged about continually, might be helpful in rounding them up.

I was afraid to see my sister, but I wanted to see her, too, so Rose and I set out for the small town where Jane had settled. We got a bit lost toward the end of the long drive, and I stopped to get directions from a bright-eyed old woman outside a house. I asked the woman if she knew where Jane lived, and she told me she was Jane, and my heart nearly jumped out of my body.

For the first few hours, I kept staring at this person I hadn't recognized. I could see now that she was my sister, and I could also see the awful distance that had grown between us.

It was a difficult visit, in many ways. Jane wasn't used to company, and I wasn't used to her, and we both worked hard to get through the day and night.

Jane came to Bedlam Farm a few months later, another tough visit. Her presence rekindled so many troubles I didn't want to see or feel. I was uncomfortable, frightened; I hadn't seen her since.

We didn't entirely lose touch. Now and then she called me and left messages. Sometimes I couldn't bear to return them; sometimes I did, and listened to endless stories about her dogs, and despaired. We wanted to reconnect, but we no longer knew each other well — so I thought. We weren't calling a brother or sister on the phone, more a stranger we'd shared a house with many years ago.

But that night, as the first storm of a nasty winter dumped a foot of snow on the farm, I dialed my sister's number and hoped that she was awake, because I wasn't sure who else I could call at that hour who would understand.

The woodstove was roaring, and Lenore was snoring; Rose was at my feet and Izzy on my lap, and I needed to talk to somebody as badly as I had ever needed anything.

I could call Paula, of course, or one of my friends, but they'd never shared such dark times with me, didn't have the same memories, hadn't felt this pain and known it for what it was.

"It's me," I said, when Jane answered the phone. If she was puzzled by the hour, she didn't say. She told me about one of her new Newfoundland pups, dogs with heart disease that she kept, sometimes for years, and watched and nurtured and loved until they died.

Telling stories about her pack, she laughed a bit, and I got angry, almost desperate. "Jane, I don't want to talk about your dogs," I said. "I'm in trouble." I hung up the phone.

There was no help for me now, I told myself. I was alone with whatever this was. A flood of familiar feelings began rolling over me, feelings I recognized from long ago, when Jane and I used to talk each other to sleep.

A moment later the phone rang. "It's me," she said. "Let's talk. What's up?" I could tell that she'd gotten the message. Something had changed. She let go of the dog talk and became my sister, loving me, worried about me, there to help me, a brave decision.

I told her I was depressed. Upset. Disoriented. I told her I was exhausted. All fall, I'd been trying to stabilize myself, and I was failing. Something old and deep was percolating up, something I couldn't bear.

And there, on the other end of the line, was my big sister. She scolded me, cautioned me, warned and guided me. She tossed all sorts of wisdom at me — stuff she'd learned in her years of twelve-stepping, perceptive insights and personal experiences mixed with psychobabble, observations, and memories.

She had been here before, done this before; she seemed ready for my call. She was soothing, comforting, wise. It was difficult, talking to Jane this way, especially at first. It wasn't a miracle. But it steadied me; somebody was out there.

I could tell Jane things I hadn't told anyone else, including my wife, my shrinks, my closest friends, because she had grown up in the same house and seen those things, too. And we had both survived them in the course of our separate but linked voyages.

Jane told me things about her life, too — the self-absorption, the overpowering world of impulses and obsession, the terrors of cocaine addiction, the ability to block out family, friends, self-interest. We traded horror stories, and in so doing found each other again.

We talked for an hour that night, for another hour the next day, and again the next night. Then once or twice a day for several weeks. We encountered problems. We had fights. We often knew what the other was going to say, and interrupted. We made each other nervous with our anger and our fear.

She soon took to calling me in the morning, then again at night. "You okay?" she'd ask.

We became each other's memory, each other's guide, as we began to piece together fragments of the puzzle that had plagued us both all our lives. I could call her in the middle of the night with ideas and memories, snippets of things I had thought or dreamed, and she could provide other pieces of this dark jigsaw.

"I didn't know these same things were in you," she said. "We've been apart for so long, I didn't know. You seemed to have figured it all out. You're married, you have a great kid, you're successful. I thought you'd escaped. Now I know."

I'd been so invested for so long in the notion of saving my sister that it was difficult to grasp how she was helping me.

We realized, slowly, over the next few weeks, that we were wrong to think we didn't know one another. We felt completely comfortable talking together, in the unquestioning way of people with a potent common experience. I didn't know how Jane spent her days or who her friends were, but I knew where we'd both come from.

I warned her that everyone in our family had abandoned everyone else, time and again. But I think we both knew that wouldn't happen now.

"This is a process," she said. "And you're in the middle of it." She used a lot of twelve-step bywords about surrendering to a higher power, taking my power back, getting my feelings validated. I disliked the vocabulary, but I didn't think the ideas were wrong.

She said she'd learned that sometimes you had to destroy the old self so that the new one could live. My old self was going down in flames; I just hoped the new one wouldn't be this disturbed.

Our conversations were interrupted continuously by Jane's instructions and reproaches to her many dogs, who needed much monitoring. "So here's what I remember," she would say, and then — "Pudge! Knock it off. Put that deer bone down." Jane fed her dogs many hearty — but, to me, revolting — things, from deer bones to turkey necks. "Sam! Whatever you're doing outside in the yard, stop it!

"You'll be okay," she'd resume, turning again to me and my miseries. "It's just feelings. It's not reality."

When I finally got myself to a therapist in Saratoga, prompted in part by my frightened wife, I talked about my drama, my past, my painful depression. And I told her the story of my sister and how she'd given herself over to me, risked her own hard-won peace of mind to help me through these dreadful days.

"You have to understand that I am not what you would call normal," Jane told me in one of our dozens of phone calls that winter. "I'm afraid of getting dressed in the morning. I'm afraid of everything. It's a part of me; I'm handicapped, and I have to live with it."

Piece by piece, argument by argument, revelation by revelation, we built a fragile platform of trust and commonality. It was not fun. It was necessary.

I reported all these conversations dutifully to Paula, a practical and grounded person who, long married to a crazy man, listened sympathetically and offered support and encouragement from the sidelines. She was always there, always on my side, but afraid. She wondered, I knew, if I could rebound from this.

I was sure of little at that point. I was sure of Paula and my daughter, Emma, and a few friends who'd drawn close.

A foolish and impulsive man sometimes, I find life has blessed me with one enduring gift: determination. When I make up my mind to do something, I usually pull it off, one way or another. I love reading about Winston Churchill and Abraham Lincoln, stubborn people, willful and focused. I often repeated Churchill's mantra: The only way through hell was to keep going through hell.

I was not going to go down this way, I decided. This was not how my story was going to end. If the only way through hell was hell, lead on.

I got up at six every morning, even when staying in bed seemed an attractive option, fed the barn cats by the back door, and walked the dogs in the woods.

I took leftover popcorn to the goats and donkey cookies to Lulu, Fanny, Jeanette, and

Jesus.

I trained Lenore.

I took a *lot* of photographs. Hundreds. Many hundreds.

I made myself three meals — healthy, well-balanced ones, suitable for a responsible diabetic.

I told the truth. If people said I looked sad, I acknowledged that I was. I tried to be open. Yes, I said, I was depressed.

I read: poems by Mary Oliver, Robert Frost, and Carl Sandburg. Thomas Merton's advice on contemplation, prayer, solitude, reflection. C. S. Lewis for inspiration; Joseph Campbell to learn about the hero's journey; Hannah Arendt on the importance of self-respect.

I took Rose out to see the sheep to remind myself of the meaning of responsibility and purpose.

I cuddled Lenore repeatedly, telling her how much I loved her, how I smiled every time I looked at her.

I agreed to all the hospice requests and took Izzy to see dying people, a reminder to keep perspective.

Izzy sat with me as I read at night, too, and used his now carefully honed healing skills to give me the love and attention so appreciated by his patients.

And every night, before bed, I called Jane. The space between us vaporized. The world seemed more in order. I liked having a big sister.

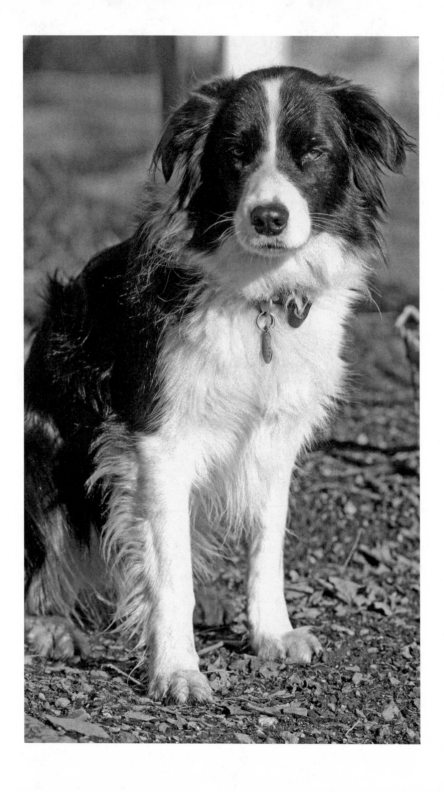

CHAPTER THIRTEEN: OFF THE BOOKS

Over the fall, word spread about Izzy and the comfort he brought. Before long, people who weren't hospice patients began to call and ask if we could come visit.

I usually said no, for several reasons. I worried about my schedule and my emotions. I found hospice visits deeply meaningful, but they also required considerable time and attention, and they extracted an emotional toll. This wasn't something I wanted to do every day, or should; it could easily become overwhelming if I didn't keep it in check. Nor did I want to give short shrift to the program by showing up for visits feeling drained, physically or emotionally.

Dealing with the terminally ill isn't for amateurs. People are often on the edge, with a great deal at stake.

The hospice program gave me access to support and guidance for myself, backup in emergencies, nurses and social workers to consult, a sort of insurance if anything went awry. Despite our careful training and good intentions, if Izzy and I went into homes whose occupants weren't part of the program, we took a gamble, and so did those families.

So when Kimberly called me in early December and asked me to visit her grandfather, who had advanced cancer, I balked. She said her family didn't believe in hospice, didn't want people coming to the house all the time.

"We can handle it ourselves," she insisted. "And we haven't given up on Pop. We are all telling him, 'Pop, don't quit on us, we need you.' And with that and God's help, he'll be around for a good long time."

I'd heard the sentiment before; it gave me pause, as well it should have. But these were friends of my neighbors, people I knew, and I couldn't see the harm of dropping by for a few minutes one afternoon. Her father was a dog lover, Kimberly said.

It was a bleak, gray, and raw day, just before dark, as Izzy and I drove to Jackson to see Joe, a retired machinist in his seventies who was enduring the late stages of colon cancer. I knew it to be a painful condition, and I'd seen how the hospice team managed it. Joe was trying to do it by himself.

He lived in an expanded trailer. Kimberly told me to look for her old Chevy pickup out front, but I didn't see a truck around when I pulled up with Izzy and knocked on the door. The trailer was covered in snow and streaked with rust. Debris was scattered around the weedy grounds — bags of trash, a stack of tires, a rusted bike.

"Hello!" I yelled. "I'm Jon!" But I didn't get out another word before a pit bull came charging around the side of the trailer. I froze and Izzy showed his teeth but stayed still as the dog came within a few feet and issued the low warning growl that can signal genuine aggression.

I pushed the trailer door open and jumped inside, pulling Izzy with me by his collar. I heard someone call the dog, which barked and then vanished. I was already wondering how I'd get Izzy and myself out of there. Hospice always checked with family members about their own dogs and cats, and asked them to confine any pets before we came, so we'd never have such an encounter.

Inside the trailer, I was taken aback by the smell — a combination of food lying around unrefrigerated, urine, and medicines. The trailer was stifling, which didn't help, warmed by a propane heater that steamed the windows.

"Hey," a weak voice called from our right. Joe, lying on a pullout sofa, was groaning and talking to himself, and I saw a bottle of whiskey on the adjacent table. "Come on in," he said. "Kim said you might be coming. I'm sorry not to get up. I'm not in great shape."

Beneath the blankets, Joe wore a thick robe. A plate of food sitting on the sofa bed had drawn the interest of a big tabby cat. Izzy noticed him before I did and gave a little growl. The cat vanished. But Izzy was unnerved for once, first by the pit bull and now by this cat.

I drew closer to the bed for a better look at Joe, close enough to be concerned that this ailing man was at home alone. He was pale and gaunt, struggling to breathe, and pain was making him grimace.

"Kim said you were bringing a dog, right? One of those therapy dogs?" Joe looked pleased for a moment, then winced and turned away. He seemed unable to focus for long. Either he'd already forgotten about Izzy or he was distracted, understandably, by his own discomfort.

Hospice volunteers are advised to go through a mental checklist about a patient's condition: Is the house clean and orderly? Does the food seem fresh? Are there smells of urine or feces? Is the medicine safely stored and administered on schedule? Is the patient clean and well groomed? Does he or she appear to be in pain? We were supposed to call in if we saw anything amiss; I rarely had.

This home, with pill bottles scattered across the kitchen, was different.

I introduced myself nevertheless and brought Izzy over. Joe seemed to appreciate the dog, and patted him briefly.

He had retired three years earlier, Joe told me, and was almost immediately stricken with cancer. It had finally laid him low, he said, after rounds of surgery, chemo, and radiation.

He had loved working in the factory, he told me. Its owners had treated him and the other workers well, until the place got taken over a few years back by some European conglomerate. It was a familiar story, upstate as everywhere: The new bosses cut benefits and hours and made work miserable. But cancer, he told me, his voice dropping to a whisper, was worse. Much worse.

Joe's eyes were runny, perhaps from a cold or just the steamy, fetid air in the trailer. I got a tissue and helped him wipe his face. In a hospice home I wouldn't be permitted to do "hands-on" treatment, but there were no rules here.

"I've about had it," he told me, not needing to be very specific. "I'm just sick of it."

But when I asked Joe if he'd thought about entering the hospice program, he waved his hand, delivered the party line. "No, I'm not about to give up, not yet. I'm a fighter. I believe in prayer. My kids and grandkids tell me not to quit. This is just a phase. I'll get back on my feet."

Kimberly came by every afternoon to help out, he said, but she had two small kids at home and worked two jobs, so he didn't want to burden her any further if he could help it.

As we were talking, she walked in, a burly brunette in her thirties, probably, carrying a sack of groceries and a small bag from the pharmacy. She thanked me profusely for coming and apologized for the condition of the place. "We don't have the money for a nurse," she said, although they did have somebody come in and clean once a week. "We do what we can."

Izzy sat by the bed for a few minutes, and Joe stroked his head now and then. But he was in too much pain to focus on the dog, and Izzy, glowering toward where he'd last seen the cat, lay down on the floor. I noticed that he didn't climb onto Joe's bed or hang around for long; he seemed as uncomfortable in the cramped space as I was.

I talked with Kimberly for a few minutes and asked her again whether hospice might not be a good idea for Joe, who looked extremely uncomfortable. Hospice would send nurses and aides without charges, I pointed out as politely as I could, and perhaps she and Joe and the trailer could use more help.

"But hospice is for people who are about to die," she said. "And we aren't ready to say good-bye to Pop."

She turned toward Joe. "Are we, Pop?" she asked, somewhat defiantly.

"No way," the weak voice came right back. "No quitters in this family."

"Right, Pop. You've got grandkids to love, right? Don't forget that. I know you won't."

Joe answered that of course he wouldn't ever forget that. Then he settled back onto his pillows with a sigh and a moan.

I didn't tell Kimberly how much I disagreed with her. I thought Joe sounded quite ready to say good-bye, but whether he was or not, he certainly didn't need to suffer this much. Why wouldn't he be willing to have less pain, cleaner surroundings, more company? This was a family that needed help but couldn't ask for it.

In any event, it was becoming clear to me

that this kind of visit was meaningless. Joe hadn't accepted his imminent death, nor had his family; as a result, they couldn't make provisions for the care he needed to be comfortable and to have a more dignified death.

All I was doing here was saying hello to a very sick man. I understood the impulse to fight a disease, but Joe had seemed, before his daughter arrived, to want to be let off the hook.

Among the many things hospice had taught me, however, was that I couldn't make decisions for other people. If Joe truly wanted to "fight," that was his decision.

Perhaps because of my own unease, Izzy seemed more uneasy than I'd seen him since we started volunteering. He paid little attention to Joe, none to Kimberly. We could both hear the pit bull barking outside, not far away. Kimberly assured me that the dog, a neighbor's, wasn't dangerous, just a bully; I should just walk quickly to my car on the way out.

So after a few minutes, Izzy and I left, and I didn't promise to come back. Joe had fallen asleep; we didn't want to wake him by saying good-bye.

Maybe I was nervous, being out here on my own. Maybe I'd passed my discomfort on to Izzy. I felt bad for this family, but decided to stick with the program. No more visits that hospice didn't set up for us. No free-lancing.

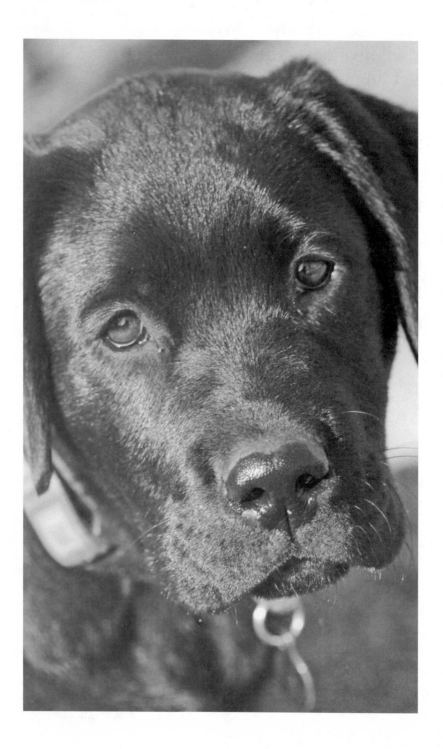

Chapter Fourteen: Puppy Love

At nine-thirty every evening, Lenore vanishes. I'm used to it now, but the first night she did it, I panicked. She's never far from me by choice.

I called her name, looked around the house, checked crates, rushed outside — shouting her name now — wondering if she was lost or stuck somewhere.

She's always responsive (especially if I'm in the kitchen), but there was no sign of her.

I searched every room in the house again, took a flashlight out back. Then I noticed the time, and it hit me.

I dashed upstairs to the bedroom, and there she was, asleep on the floor, ready for dreamland but still too little to jump onto the bed. She was waiting for me to come help her up.

"Hey, sweetie," I said, leaning down. I put one hand under her rump and lifted her up; her tail started wagging and she chewed on my face a bit, then fell asleep in my arms. Lenore was not anxious about my dropping her. Lenore was not anxious about anything.

She curled up on the pillow and was snoring before I could leave the room. "What a goofball," I said with a laugh, scratching her nose; she yawned but didn't wake up.

I was struck once more by the ability of a well-trained Lab to make herself comfortable in any setting.

My border collies rarely leave my side while I'm awake; Rose keeps hoping for work, at any hour. I can't imagine Izzy going off to bed by himself, either. Lenore, comfortable in her own skin, had no qualms about padding upstairs at bedtime. She knew I'd be along eventually, and meanwhile, why waste a perfectly good chance to doze?

As much as any dog I've had, Lenore is a creature of light and laughter. If Izzy could go into one home after another and bring comfort and peace to the dying, Lenore could come into my own home, in the midst of a miserable time, and make me smile, almost every time I encountered her.

She would have been a gift at any time. That winter, she was a treasure. Lenore was doing for me what Izzy was doing for the patients he was seeing, connecting to me in an instinctive way.

Her love was vast, oceanic, not only for me but for every living thing, and some inanimate ones, too. She had heaps of personality, was curious and alert and playful. The love affair we had going reminded me almost hourly of why I love dogs — choosing them, living with them, training them — and why, in that shadowy winter, my acquiring this source of light was a good instinct. Dogs do all kinds of things for people, I was learning yet again.

Through the day, Lenore looked up from her sleep, or from whatever she was chewing on, and noticed me; her dark eyes widened and her tail thumped, and she came tumbling over, wriggling into my lap, crawling up onto the sofa, or snuggling with me in bed. She happily licked my nose or burrowed her big soft head into my hand. She loved to have me rub her belly. She enjoyed my habit of reciting Poe's poetry to her, though probably it was just the sound of my voice she liked, since she was equally enthusiastic when I called her Lenore the Whore — the playful epithet I'd awarded her for being so prodigally generous with her affections. I could hardly believe Labradors' willingness to turn themselves over, body and soul, to anybody carrying a biscuit, but it

215

was also what I loved about the breed.

Outside, Lenore watched me closely on our walks, running over to ascertain if I had a treat, to try to entice me into throwing something she could fetch. She had a mischievous twinkle, and a minor rebellious streak. If she smelled something sufficiently gross, she tilted her head when I ordered her away and obeyed perhaps fifty percent of the time. I couldn't be as stern and consistent as I'd been with Izzy or Rose; she was simply too ridiculously cute.

She was well adapted to the bleak days I'd been enduring. Unlike people, she won't expect you to be chipper or responsive. She will love you as intensely when you're down as when you're happy. It makes no difference to her, as long as she gets fed. It helps if you have treats, but even that is negotiable.

Lenore was by no means a perfect dog; there is no such creature. She ate all kinds of disgusting stuff: chicken droppings and deer scat, dead things in the woods, pens and Ziploc bags, socks, twigs. Then she'd lie in front of Izzy and Rose while they chewed their rawhide, waiting intently for them to lose interest.

When I go into the kitchen now, I have a black shadow. She doesn't beg or jump, she waits and watches. Once in a while, a bit of something falls, and she pounces.

Sometimes this is useful, as when I dropped half a dozen eggs on the floor and they splattered all over the place. Lenore, astonished at first, quickly realized that these splotches were food and was beside herself. She walked in the goo, rolled in it, licked up every single bit of yolk, white, and shell. By the time I got out the paper towels and spray cleaner, there wasn't much left to clear off the floor. Lenore, however, was a sticky, foul mess requiring a dunk in the bathtub.

I'm not her only fan. When Annie's husband, Joe, heads into Salem to go to the hardware store, he stops by the farm to pick up Lenore. He has standing approval to take her on his travels because he's crazy about her; also because these excursions help socialize her and expose her to all sorts of people; also because she loves to go along.

"I've got Lenore," he yells from the back door as Lenore bounds out of the house into his truck and spends the next half hour enthusiastically greeting strangers and customers in the store and on the street.

A master ride-along dog, she accompanies me on photo shoots. While Izzy curls up in the backseat and barely moves, Lenore sticks her head out the window to observe me. She never jumps out of the car, except for that time in front of a Chinese restaurant in Glen Falls when a teenager dropped her take-out egg roll onto the sidewalk.

Lenore squeezed out of the car window in a millisecond, and had wolfed down the egg roll before the girl even realized it was gone. I offered to buy her another one, but she cuddled with Lenore instead, cooing, "Awwww, puppy." Lenore can get away with anything.

Dogs react so differently to humans. When somebody comes to the house, Rose runs to find me and sit by my side; she won't go off with a stranger, or even with most of the people she knows well.

Izzy will go easily with an acquaintance, but not with a stranger. Given a choice, he'd rather hang around with me.

Lenore really couldn't care less, and it's that quality — her blithely genial, loving (and hungry) nature — that I prize most about her.

Lenore brings light into my life, to the farm, into the lives of the other dogs — to almost anyone who drifts into her consciousness. I needed a dog like that.

Four weeks after I brought this pup home, I took her out into the woods for a camping weekend. Maria and her husband, Bill, helped us tote our gear. It was a slightly ambitious undertaking for a dog Lenore's age; I wasn't sure how she would react. Could she handle the mile-long hike in to the cabin? (Could I?) Would she run off? Could she be quiet and calm in an environment where there wasn't much to do, or much space to do it in? Mostly, I intended to read, take photos, hike, and sit around gazing at the fire. Would a young puppy be annoying? There would be no crate, no way to confine her — would her housebreaking training hold up?

The big problem on the hike in, it emerged, was that Lenore appointed herself Official Greeter of the Merck Forest Preserve. Whenever she saw another hiker or camper, she went bounding over, all excited, tail waving. Several families with kids gave her lots of hugs and squeals, and she would happily have trotted off with them if I hadn't called to her and made sure she stayed close by.

Once off the busy-ish main trail, she settled down, tagged along, and had no trouble walking the distance. She loved the cabin, as it turned out, was delighted to sit out under the stars with me, happy to watch me cook. She eagerly came along on several short hikes, then gnawed on a log before falling asleep.

At bedtime, I put her next to me on the bunk, and she wriggled up against my sleeping bag and, worn out, barely moved an inch all night. She went outside to eliminate, and graciously accompanied me to the outhouse. She got the idea of coming along to the firewood shed, and happily trotted beside me. I was a bit nervous, since I couldn't see this jet-black creature in the dark and didn't even want to think about her wandering off in a forest filled with coyotes and bobcats.

But she didn't wander; she was a perfect companion. Having two days and nights with Lenore out in the Vermont woods was lovely, a perfect way for a person and a dog to bond. There was no one but me for her to pay attention to, except for the occasional hiker trekking nearby. I took advantage of the opportunity to hand-feed her, and train her, and take her for walks along a beautiful ridge.

I think any dog — but particularly a working and hunting breed like a Lab — could have picked up on my vibes that weekend: appreciation for the beauty of the place, the sweetness of solitude and stillness, the pleasure of reading a good book by a good stove, the sense of serenity. Lenore seemed to understand. I would look up occasionally and see her staring out at the valley below, just as I was.

Two days later, we hiked back to the car, Lenore walking proudly alongside me. It was a tonic to spend a couple of days and nights with so simple and loving a companion; every camper ought to have one.

She's woven herself into my daily routine now. Her day unofficially begins around five a.m., when she stirs, creeps up to put her head on my shoulder, nibbles on my chin, then goes back to sleep. It's the first of many times in the course of a day that Lenore makes me smile.

Around six, I usually turn on the light and read for a few minutes, get up, shower, and dress. Rose is usually sitting at the foot of the bed, Izzy curled up underneath it, Lenore jammed in against my back or my neck, wherever is warmest.

Coming out of the bathroom and putting my boots on is the signal for the dogs to bound down the stairs and head for the door, rush up the slope next to the farm-house, and do their stuff.

When they come in, I feed them. Meals are something the border collies can usually take or leave, but Lenore is almost beside herself at the prospect of breakfast, wiggling and waggling, nearly collapsing head first into the food bowl when I set it on the floor.

It's almost comical to watch Rose and Lenore eat. Usually, I have to call Rose two or three times from her perch at the living room window, where she is studiously observing the sheep. Lenore has usually gulped her food down before Rose has taken her first delicate, unenthusiastic nibble.

Around seven, we go for our first walk on the woodland path. Lenore, I think, may imagine she's a border collie; she bounds after Rose and Izzy as they rocket off into the woods. But she's not nearly as swift. She runs as far as she can, then turns back; walking beside me is her second-best choice.

She will veer off to prowl the woods for disgusting stuff to eat and roll in, but she never runs away. To make sure it stays that way, I drop a treat on the ground every few minutes to keep her interested in me and focused on the walk.

At some point during the morning walk, we do our obedience drills — sit down, lie, stay. These grounding exercises are critical, a major reason Lenore is as calm and well behaved as she is. I try to be disciplined about taking her through these training exercises two or three times a day, briefly and with encouragement.

When we get back to the farmhouse, I put a dab of peanut butter on three rawhide strips and give one to each of the dogs in the front yard. Rose runs off into the garden with hers, out of sight. Izzy sniffs and stares until he's ready to chew. Lenore's body gyrates with gratitude and she settles on the porch with glee.

I come inside, make myself some breakfast, phone Paula if she's not in residence, wait for Annie to show up and help with the barnyard chores. Then I fire up the woodstove and go to work, after opening the front door so the three dogs can come tearing in.

Lenore has effortlessly taken over the role of lead literary dog; she embodies all the qualities of a first-class writing assistant. She is not restless; in fact, a bomb could go off in the front yard and, if she's deep in sleep, she'll barely notice. She crawls beneath my desk, happy to serve as inspiration or comfort, and there she remains until I turn the computer off.

The border collies never really stop investigating things. Rose checks on the sheep; Izzy moves to the window to see what's driving by. When Lenore rests, however, she gives it her full attention. I like working with her nearby, present but unobtrusive; it settles me. The days pass with this quiet routine.

We walk again in the late morning, and again after lunch. In warm weather, we might herd sheep or run with the ATV. In cold weather, more lying around the stove, more work for me.

In the afternoon we throw the ball, walk through the barn, check on the farm animals. Then feeding time for the dogs.

By dark, they're done. Lenore patrols the house, collecting chewbones and plush toys, gnawing on them fitfully, but she's losing interest. She finds me and either curls up near my feet or hops up next to me on the sofa, to get her belly scratched, or to put her head on my knee. I love everybody, she seems to be telling me, but I know I'm your dog.

If I stay up later than she finds appropriate, she will climb up the stairs and await my help. It's bedtime.

She's a good dog to have in the winter, a warm dog. Two or three times during the night, she crawls up alongside my face, nuzzles me, gives me a lick or two. I kiss her on the nose. As much as any creature or thing, Lenore has helped draw me out of the shadows, toward the light.

Those smiles she generated added up,

helped pull me out of myself. Her unquestioning love was always there, always soothing, always reassuring. Her funny stunts and joyous personality reminded me that there was life beyond the shadows, and she and I might tiptoe there together.

In that way, this unassuming, warmhearted creature did me a good turn. She connected with me, touched an instinct in me, and the instinct told me things would be okay.

Lenore, it turned out, was a therapy pup.

In January, when she was nearly six months old, I took Lenore to her first hospice meeting. Jeff Meyer, the vet, agreed she had the temperament for this kind of work — she was gentle, loving, trustworthy around people. The meeting was held at the county office annex in Fort Edward.

Izzy came along, too, of course. If I'd shown up at a hospice event without him, I think there's a good chance I'd have been turned away.

When we arrived, about a dozen people had gathered around a conference table; on a separate table sat a pile of doughnuts and cookies, the universal snack for budget-conscious nonprofits.

Lenore bounded into the room and excitedly rushed over to greet the other volunteers. She put her paws on their knees and jumped up to kiss them, her tail whipping a mile a minute. "Off!" I said sharply, still working to train her out of overexuberance. Then she began exploring every inch of the room for crumbs, bits of doughnuts, and other food left behind from a hundred other meetings. She sniffed the stack of cookies and started to approach the table, but I headed her off.

Izzy, meanwhile, trotted over to Keith Mann, the chief of volunteers, who'd led our training. Izzy was delighted to hang out with Keith, who always stashed a few biscuits for him in his pocket.

I kept Lenore on a leash. Whenever Izzy moved, she got up, and I made her lie down. I took her around the room, and she was happy to see everybody, enthusiastic. I did a few obedience exercises with her, just for practice. Then she slept, but she hopped up when somebody entered or left the room, or moved.

Watching her closely, and watching Izzy, I was struck by how different these two dogs were. I'd taken Izzy to a dozen such meetings and never once had to correct or monitor him. He usually circled the table once, offering everybody his head to pat, and then curled up under the table or off in a corner.

Once in a while he came up to visit with Keith, who patted him while he spoke; then Izzy vanished again.

As I listened to the volunteers, with their easy humor and gentle natures, talk about their experiences with various patients, I was still keeping an eye on my dogs. It was instructive.

As the meeting ended, I picked Lenore up and hugged her, giving her nose a squishy kiss. She returned the favor. "You lug," I said.

On our way out, she detoured to extract a bit of cookie embedded beneath one of the conference-table legs.

I was learning some things. I had turned myself over to the process of psychotherapy by now and thought I was beginning to emerge from the shadows. As much as any other being, except perhaps my wife and my outspoken shrink, Lenore had helped me, mostly by simply existing.

I was grateful to her. I owed her.

But what precisely did I owe her? I wondered, as Izzy bounded ahead of me and sat by the car door, anticipating me, as usual, and Lenore scoured the parking lot for something to sniff or devour.

I owed her the right to be herself, I recognized as we drove home — not a clone of

Izzy, not some other version of what I or anyone else thought a dog ought to be.

One of the biggest lessons I was learning that winter was to separate my own life and concerns from the problems and lives of others. Easy to say, not easy to do. But here was a chance to put the principle into practice.

Lenore wasn't really a good candidate for a hospice dog, at least not yet. She wasn't as gentle or intuitive as Izzy. Her instinct was to smother everybody with affection, a great quality in a dog, but not for hospice work, where people's last days often required that they be approached with exquisite sensitivity, something Izzy had but Lenore didn't.

I could — and would — train her not to jump on people. I would train her to be calm and appropriate. But I didn't want to subject her to the pressure of being as tranquil as Izzy, nor could I subject dying patients to a dog as enthusiastic and boisterous as Lenore. I knew how easy it was to make dogs crazy when you tried to change their essential natures. Izzy's hospice work played to his natural strengths. Lenore had her own great traits, but different ones.

So I decided I'd let Lenore be Lenore. I booted her out of hospice training, and when we got home that evening, we went up to the bedroom and I wrapped my arms

228

around her and thanked her profusely for being the dog she was. She thumped her tail, chewed on my nose, and fell asleep.

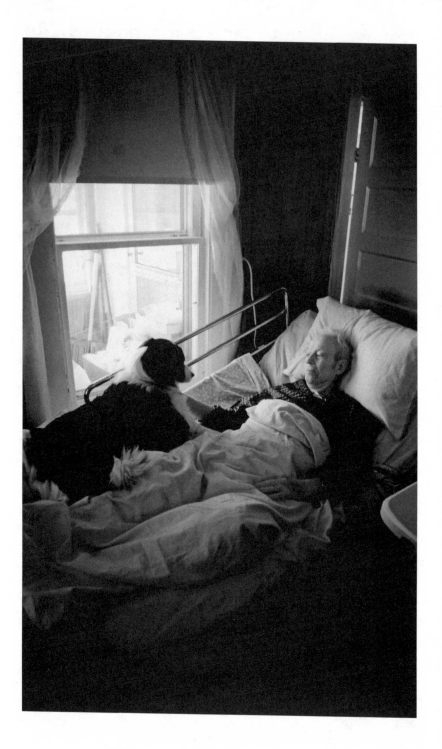

Chapter Fifteen:
Glen

Glen leaned back on his pillows, reached over to stroke Izzy's head, and for the umpteenth time began the story of how he got his first pickup truck. We both chuckled.

Glen was in pain from his prostate cancer, and knew he was close to death, but he retained a capacity for laughter. This story was becoming comical, a standing joke.

He'd been trying to tell Izzy and me about the truck, and how he used it to haul logs all over New York State and Vermont and eastern Canada, for a week now. Sometimes he had to stop to take his medicine or talk to the nurse; sometimes he had to change position, or he fell asleep.

"When I was born," he would start, "I had what they used to call a club foot. My parents were poor and had to give me up. They couldn't afford a boy on the farm who couldn't work. So my grandparents took me, and I did all right. I was okay.

They took care of me."

His grandfather made him a splint for his bad foot, and with it he could work. "My parents wanted me back," he went on. "But my grandparents said no, they couldn't have me back. It was okay. I did all right."

Working on his grandparents' dairy farm one day, Glen saw a milk trucker pull in early in the morning — and there was born the inspiration to try to drive a truck himself, and maybe, one day, own one.

That was as far as Glen ever got in the story, though. To hear the rest, I'd have to be patient.

Glen had spent most of his life in this sparsely settled corner of the eastern Adirondacks. The drive north to his house, though it was in the same county, took me close to two hours. It was an exotic trip, through a living museum of a lost America: crumbling, shuttered towns, trailer parks and closed motels, failed businesses whose glory days were far in the past. It was eerie to drive through so much natural beauty and so much severe poverty.

Glen's tiny house, sided with white aluminum, had a staggering view of the glorious mountain range that cuts through New York State. Elsewhere, that view would be worth hundreds of thousands of dollars. Not here.

Inside, lying next to a window that abutted a small glassed-in porch, Glen lay in a hospital bed. He was a slight man, with white hair and wide blue eyes. From the pictures around the house, showing him as a young man, I could see that he'd always been small and thin, yet strong — the muscles of his arms were still taut.

His cancer was advancing rapidly, spreading to his bones; his heart was failing, and soon his brain would, too. He wasn't expected to live much longer. His wife had died suddenly six months earlier, his devoted dog a few years before that. Now Glen was being cared for by devoted in-laws, and by hospice.

Getting assigned to Glen was not a casual matter, for me or for the hospice administrators. He was the kind of patient a volunteer could get attached to. "You're going to love him, and he's going to love you and Izzy, so we have to be careful," Keith Mann cautioned.

The dynamics of hospice care were very involved; I was getting used to the idea that nothing was taken for granted. The stakes — the way somebody died — were high, and no detail too trivial for the staff to consider.

They knew me by now, and knew what to

watch out for — that I would get too involved with Glen, and be too deeply affected by his death. In hospice, volunteers are monitored almost as carefully as the patients. It's never easy to see someone die, but some situations are more demanding than others; the staff knew this one would be difficult for me.

Unlike some of the patients we'd seen, Glen was alert, a raconteur full of memories and country tales. And he was a dog lover through and through. His own dog, a collie-shepherd mix he named Pal, had been his constant companion on the road for years; he would grasp the meaning of a good dog like Izzy.

Glen needed to talk about his life, the hospice social worker told me, and I loved to listen to the kinds of stories he could tell me. He'd welcome a chance to reconnect with a dog. It was a good deal all around.

Still, as I drove north through the Adirondacks, mesmerized by the lonesome beauty of abandoned cabins and other ghosts, I went through the hospice mantra to prepare myself: You are there to listen, not to cheer anybody up, although sometimes that amounts to the same thing. This man isn't going to get better; he's going to die, probably soon. As soon as you get to know him, he's likely to decline further, and then his energy and spirit will turn inward and he might not even recognize you. Leave your own stuff at the door. It's okay to be quiet. Make sure he has the space and comfort he needs to do what he needs to do.

Glen was as advertised — lucid, likable, as eager to tell stories as I was to hear them. He predictably adored Izzy, who almost immediately sprang lightly onto the hospital bed and lay down beside him, reminding him of his companion, Pal, who'd ridden with him in logging trucks sixteen hours a day, six days a week, for many years. "A million miles, I might say," said Glen, proudly. "Give or take, give or take." He showed us a small wood carving of Pal that a lumberjack friend had whittled for him, a treasured memento.

To me, Glen's life was exotic, something out of a bygone, sepia-toned America. He was matter-of-fact about it, though. "No point in lying now," Glen told me more than once, not that he seemed likely to lie at any point.

He spent his whole youth with his grandparents, but later went to see the parents who'd sent him away. "I made peace with them," he said. "It was hard times for everybody, and everybody did the best they could. No point in feeling bad about it."

Always poor, somehow — details would have to wait, I guessed — he did buy his own logging truck and spent decades riding around the forests of the Northeast.

He married a poor farm girl, Pearlie, and they had a son, born with cerebral palsy. Glen never went to school, or took a vacation, or bought a single thing he didn't absolutely need. You could view his life as mean, disadvantaged, but in his view he'd had a great life, filled with the pride and freedom of running his own business, with the love of a family and good friends, and "well, just about everything I ever needed. Yeah."

If money was short, Glen might take on a Sunday run. Otherwise, Sundays were for him and his son, Louis; they went out for ice cream cones every week, without fail.

He spent the other six days driving from logging fields to sawmills, with only Pal for company. Lunch, he told me confidentially, was "two cans of beans with some meat in it" — one can for him, one for Pal. Or he might stop at a diner for two hot dogs.

This was a sidekick who deserved such rewards. More than once Pal had run off hungry bears who showed up when Glen broke for lunch.

When he recalled Pal's fidelity and companionship on those long, lonely drives, Glen's voice cracked. He kept the little carving close by his bed.

"My dog wanted to chase things, sure," he said. "But he never ran off, not once. Yeah."

Our love of dogs aside, we could hardly have been more different. "What do you do?" Glen asked me several times. I write books about dogs, animals, and rural life, I told him.

Yes, but what do you do?

I have a farm, I told him. Sheep, goats, a few cows and chickens.

Do you send your animals to market? he wanted to know.

No, I said. I keep them and write about them.

But how do your make your living?

Eventually, this became another of our running jokes. A hardworking man for more than half a century who wasn't much of a reader, how could he grasp that someone could pay the bills by hanging around dogs and other animals? After a while, I just told him I did hospice work.

It was just as hard for me to imagine riding around all day with logs on a truck.

"Did they ever fall off?" I asked once, needling him a bit. He was so conscientious about his truck that I wondered if he'd ever cut corners, had mishaps.

"Oh, yeah," he said, through a wide grin. "In the old days, you didn't have to put chains on 'em, you just piled 'em on in the mill and drove around. Once in a while, one of 'em would fall off."

What did you do then, I wondered.

He winked. "If I could, I'd just hit the gas and keep going."

Our visits quickly took on their own rhythms. En route, I stopped at Dunkin' Donuts for coffee and at a local market for some fresh flowers before Izzy and I made the long drive north.

When we opened the porch door, Glen could see us through the window and eagerly waved us through. He always asked if I wanted water or something to eat.

Often, I urged John or Ann, Glen's brother-in-law and his wife, who were caring for him, to go out, do some errands or chores. Hospice called this "respite," and this couple needed some. John usually dashed out to feed his chickens.

Glen spent his days in the shag-carpeted living room, which was crammed with medical equipment, furniture, towels, bottles of medicine, the accessories and contraptions of the chronically ill. At night, John moved him into his bedroom, where he spent a restless night.

I don't think either of them had known a good night's sleep in months. John was attentive, conscientious, uncomplaining; Glen had been good to him all through his life, he said, and now when Glen needed it, he was going to be there for him.

It was a tough space for Izzy to work in, because it was so small and crowded. He sprang carefully up onto the foot of the hospital bed and snuggled next to Glen, who put a hand on his head. He had to sandwich himself between Glen and the safety bars on either side — not much room for a good-sized dog.

I took many photographs of Glen and Izzy together, great friends from their first encounter. (The family had asked me to record this time.)

Glen was crazy about Izzy, although I soon realized that the advancing cancer had made Glen very sensitive to touch. If Izzy even leaned into him too hard, I could tell by Glen's wince that it caused pain. Yet Glen was much too polite to complain, so I had to be vigilant and make sure Izzy didn't get too close.

After the first visit or two, Izzy himself seemed to understand. He lay down, put his head into Glen's hand, stayed still. If I got up — to go to the bathroom, bring Glen some water, answer the phone — Izzy remained glued to the spot.

Having Izzy there invariably reminded Glen of Pal, and when he remembered Pal he cried a bit, the only time he showed much emotion.

"He even looks like Pal," he said, weeping as Izzy went into his drill. Sometimes he cried so hard I had to bring him some tissues.

"I'm sorry," he said. "I don't usually tear up like this, but I just lost my wife, Pearlie, last summer, and now, seeing this sheepdog, I can't help but think of Pal. He was such a good dog."

I enjoyed the stillness of the simple house, where the only sound was the hissing of Glen's oxygen supply. He'd balked, initially, at having those plastic tubes inserted into his nostrils, but as his breathing became more labored, he relented.

I sat in a chair on the other side of the bed, looking out at his spectacular mountain view and the soft light coming through the window. It was peaceful, though increasingly interrupted by reality — Glen coughed up blood, had bursts of pain, suffered indigestion and incontinence.

He told me his nights were getting rougher — more pain, less sleep, disturbing dreams. "Won't be long, will it? Yeah?" he would ask at some point during every visit.

He'd been suffering for a long time, first with heart disease, then the cancer. He had a pacemaker, and his cancer was spreading despite several surgeries. He didn't want any more of that. "Please," he begged me. "No more operations, no machines keeping me going. Nothing stuck in my arms or down my throat." That was up to him, I said.

My role was never quite clear to Glen, who seemed to assume I was some sort of hospice official who might be able to tell him when and how he would die. I said I was just a volunteer there to give the family a break, and bring Izzy and keep him company. I doubt he ever quite believed me.

He was wary of talking to doctors and nurses, fearing he might end up in a hospital, getting another operation, or be sent to a nursing home. But he did confide in me and told me of his confusion, worsening pain, and weakening limbs. He said he'd overheard a relative talking on the phone, and that's how he knew he had — and he whispered the words — "stage-four cancer."

"Jon," he whispered to me one afternoon, as he and Izzy were cuddled on the bed, "I'm done." But then he launched bravely into one of his stories.

He talked about the time, up by the Canadian border, that a thief broke into his truck to steal cigarettes. The guy emerged from the truck with Pal hanging off one arm. He pulled out a pistol and was about to plug Pal, until Glen begged him, "Please, don't shoot my dog." The robber left, without the cigarettes, and without shooting Pal. The thought of that near calamity still brought Glen to tears, decades later.

He never complained about his illness, or talked very much about dying. His old dog was the vehicle through which he could face love and loss. And Izzy was the way to get to the dog.

I'd been around hospice long enough, by this point, to know that when patients cried, it wasn't always about the things they said they were crying about. One of the benefits Izzy could offer was to help people access the swirling emotions around death.

The Pal stories — and we heard quite a few over those cold, windswept days — were special for other reasons, too: They painted an eloquent picture of the role a dog can play. This one added a rich dimension to what could have been a lonely, solitary life.

Glen used to get up every morning at

three, he said. When he got to his truck —
he bought a new Ford every three years, he
told me proudly, with the biggest heater
made — Pal was waiting for him by the
door.

"You know, Jon," he would confide, "you
can always turn the heat down, but if you
don't have a big heater and you're up by the
Canadian border in January, you can't always turn it up.

It was because of Pal, he said, that he met
his wife. She was hitchhiking to work near
Ticonderoga and Pal barked, so he pulled
over, Glen said.

"Pal loved her from the start. And I
thought, 'Well, if I don't marry her, he'll
leave me and I'll lose my dog.' " A few weeks
later, when he came to pick Pearl up for a
date, her father was waiting for him with a
rifle, and fired the gun straight into the air.

"What did you do that for?" Glen asked,
scared out of his wits.

"So you'd see it," her father said. He went
on to announce that he'd rather see Pearl in
her grave than married to Glen, but she married him anyway, and they were together for
nearly sixty years.

He told me, too, how Pal ran into a neighbor's barn a few years back and apparently
ate some rat poison. He collapsed on the

floor of the vet's office, where Glen had rushed him. "That's how my dog Pal died," Glen told me, in tears again.

I came to look forward to those drives, getting my coffee, pulling over to take photos of bait shops and ancient barns on the way, then steering in to Glen's house, where I always got a warm welcome.

Friends, neighbors, and town officials stopped by to check on things, too, including the head of the town highway department, who made Glen's house a part of his daily rounds.

One Saturday afternoon in our third week — Glen was alert, but weakening — when Izzy hopped onto the bed, something was different. As I watched, Glen seemed to slip into a deep unconsciousness, almost a coma. Ann and I looked at each other; she saw it, too.

We had seen this turn before, Izzy and I. We met hospice patients who were alert, comfortable, talkative — until, inevitably, there came a point where the illness worsened, the body weakened, the pain increased, and so did the medication to relieve it.

This was the period hospice workers called "actively dying," when patients quieted, turned inward, and their bodies began to shut down. There might still be moments of consciousness and alertness, but fewer. It was a clear signal that the person was entering the final phase. Often, this development caused a patient to focus more on himself, less on visitors, even if the visitor in question was a bighearted dog.

Izzy sensed this change, too, often transferring his focus from the patient to the family. But I also noticed over time that he appeared drained when that happened. I couldn't know what Izzy was thinking, but it sometimes seemed that he was discouraged, the way search-and-rescue dogs can be when they can't find victims still alive in disasters. Comforting hospice patients had become Izzy's work, and I wondered if he didn't see their moving away from him, their dying, as a failure.

On this afternoon, Izzy stared at Glen intently, then looked at me. He gently jumped down from the bed. Ann kneeled and began to pray.

We came to see Glen often after that, but he never fully regained consciousness, never took another meal, never told another story.

When Izzy came onto the bed, Glen sometimes responded, but usually didn't, so Izzy would hop off and turn his attention to Ann, who sat by Glen's side, holding his hand. She told Glen the Lord was ready whenever he was, that he should let go, that his son would be well cared for, that he had suffered enough.

Glen was not a "church man," he had informed me, but had agreed to let Ann baptize him, just in case he needed that to be with Pearl in heaven. "I figure it can't hurt," he had said. "And I would hate to finally get up there, if that's where I'm going, and get barred because I wasn't baptized." So Ann baptized him with a sprinkling of water and some prayers one morning, just before Izzy and I arrived.

Izzy could join in the spirit of Ann's devotion, putting his head on her knee or lying by her feet as she kneeled. More and more, I noticed, these two had formed an attachment. He rarely took his eyes off her, and Ann always wanted to know where Izzy was. His work had changed.

Mine had, too. I tried now to be useful to the family, who were obviously strained and exhausted.

I was in awe of the strength and dedication of these families, and also by the loneliness that frequently engulfed them as friends, acquaintances, even other family members stayed away. Ann and John cleaned up blood, changed diapers, monitored oxygen and drugs, cooked meals, cleaned and shopped and ran errands for Glen, while also coping with the details of their own homes and children. Their lives had been suspended by Glen's illness, yet their lives went on. They were weary, confused sometimes, grateful for even an hour out. They perked up visibly when the hospice nurses, aides, volunteers, and social workers came by.

Often, the families need to talk. John and Ann spoke with me about Glen, their lives and experiences with him, their feelings about his life and death. They told stories, traded anecdotes about how hard he'd worked to take care of his disabled son, Louis, who had moved recently to a group home when Glen became too ill to care for him. They talked about his generosity, his uncomplaining nature. He had helped them so many times, they recalled, and now it was their turn. They hoped his passing would be swift and merciful. They hoped Jesus was waiting for him.

I worked to keep some boundaries around this relationship, which had grown increasingly affecting. Following Keith's instructions, I didn't go every day; three or four times a week was enough. I didn't bring food, though I did continue to bring fresh flowers to brighten the room. I reminded myself each morning that Glen wasn't going to miraculously revive or recover.

One Wednesday in January, John called me at home and said that Glen was failing. The hospice nurse had just been by; Glen wasn't expected to last the day.

"Do you want us to come?" I asked.

"Please," he said. "Ann and I want you and Izzy to be there."

We made the drive up to the Adirondacks in a little over an hour. I was prepared to wave my hospice ID at any state trooper who stopped me for speeding.

I'd gotten to know Glen better than any of the people we'd met. I loved his stories of logging days, his warmth and spirit. I was determined to help him have a good death, just as he'd had a good life.

He had, for me, come to embody the hospice idea: that death was sad, but it didn't have to be depressing. Pain could be relieved, family could be nearby, people could control the way they left the world, with dignity and autonomy. Glen was dying the way he wished to, and we were helping him.

When we arrived, around noon, the hospital bed had been moved into the center of the living room; Glen no longer needed the view. The hospice aides and nurse had already come, and Glen had been bathed and dressed in fresh flannel pajamas.

John was sitting quietly in the kitchen, reading, doing a few chores, thinking about the man who had taken him to buy his first car. "He was a good friend to me," he said. "Always."

I could see that Glen's condition had changed just since our visit two days earlier. His eyes were closed, he showed no sign of being conscious at all, and he was breathing slowly and heavily. His hands were cold.

Izzy went to him for perhaps thirty seconds. Then, as had become his custom in recent days, he left Glen and went to Ann, dropping by her feet.

"Oh, Izzy," she said, embracing him. "Thank you for coming. I hope the Lord takes Glen today, he's ready and has suffered enough. I hope he goes to be with his Pearlie." Izzy pressed his head against Ann's knee and stayed there for a good fifteen minutes.

Ann prayed for Glen and held his hand. I spoke to Glen and read him a few Carl Sandburg poems — "Tall Timber" and "The Great Proud Wagon Wheels Go On" and "Proud Torsos" — poems that seemed to relate to his life.

I'm not always at ease with conventional

religious observance, but I felt close to Ann, so when she asked if I would pray with her, I was happy to sit next to her and bow my head. She asked God to give Glen the strength to go, asked Him to ease Glen's journey, to welcome him home, to reunite him with Pearl, to recognize the good and honest way he'd lived his life.

Whenever Ann prayed, Izzy stared at her intently and they seemed to almost fuse, these two loving spirits. Glen was no longer conscious of Izzy, nor was Izzy paying much attention, as if Glen was no longer truly there and Izzy knew that their connection had concluded. There was someone else who needed his comfort now.

Ann worried about Izzy, too. When Glen didn't respond to him, she hugged him. "You seem so sad, Izzy," she crooned. "Glen is leaving us soon but you did everything you could. Don't be sad." He gazed at her and offered his paw.

I noticed that Glen's breathing was getting slower, deeper. He seemed to be almost visibly shutting down. Ann had trouble looking at him and asked me how he was doing. John suddenly said he had to go to the bank, and he wouldn't be long; I told him to go. He couldn't bear to see Glen pass, Ann said.

A little after two-thirty, with Ann praying

and holding Glen's hand with her right hand, Izzy's paw with her left, I noticed that Glen no longer seemed to be breathing. I leaned forward to time his breathing as I'd been taught. Two minutes passed without a breath, and I got up and hugged Ann.

"Ann," I said. "I think Glen is gone. He's not breathing."

She nodded, squeezed his hand, asked God to take him home. Then she leaned over to cry and embrace Izzy for a long time.

I closed Glen's eyes, pulled the blanket over his face. Ann asked if I could call hospice. In the kitchen, I dialed the emergency number we'd been given; a hospice nurse said she was on her way. Then John came home and we told him Glen had died, and he nodded.

Ann asked me to help pick out the clothes Glen would be buried in. We chose his good brown suit, black shoes, a white shirt, and a musty old tie. I set the wood carving of Pal atop the stack of garments, along with a photo of his wife and son. We turned off the oxygen machine and waited for the nurse and the undertaker.

Somewhere during these moments of preparation, Izzy found a quiet corner and curled up there. He seemed drained and despondent. I take care not to attribute human emotions to animals, but it was hard not to believe that he was dejected, as if he'd failed somehow. The most cheerful of creatures, he seemed exhausted. Eventually, he came out and climbed onto the other bed Glen had used.

Busy with other things, I glanced over at him from time to time. The hospice staff arrived and took over, and then the undertaker appeared with his assistant, and people were scurrying around the house, preparing Glen for his final trip from home. But Ann was worried about Izzy and came over to hug him.

It seemed time to go. Glen had died; there was plenty of help on the scene. We said our good-byes and I slipped out the door. Glen's family had to deal with this loss in their own way, and I didn't want to intrude on that.

I felt all sorts of things, pulling away from that simple house on the hill for the last time. I was proud of Izzy; I was proud of me.

We'd helped Glen to die. We helped his family deal with his death. I was grateful for the training that prepared me, so that I could be helpful. I didn't mess anything up, which is always nice. We did our jobs.

Everybody told Izzy he had found his calling. Perhaps he had led me to mine, too. It was impossible, I knew, to separate one's own history and needs from the things we did for others. I knew that my hospice work was as much for my own benefit as for anybody who was dying. It was, in some way, healing.

I enjoyed being told that I was doing something valuable, something a lot of people didn't feel comfortable doing. I enjoyed having a dog who could do it with the intuition, love, and skill that Izzy had.

I found it meaningful to know a man like Glen, like the others we'd met through hospice, and to be permitted into their lives at this most intimate moment.

To come so close to death is to also be close to life, to rebirth and renewal.

Four days later, John called to ask us to Glen's memorial service, at a funeral home in a nearby town.

When we arrived, Izzy lay by the casket for a long time, then attached himself to Ann. I marveled at the connection between them, their understanding of each other.

I told her that Glen had been unable to finish telling me the story of his pickup. She laughed, said she'd heard it a million times and would be happy to finish it.

Milk trucks arrived daily at his grandparents' farm, she said, and one of the drivers, seeing the boy's awe, took him for a ride. Glen realized that this was something he could do, even with a bad foot: He could have his own business. At first, as a teenager, he borrowed pickups and hauled things for people. Small jobs — but he saved enough money for his own first truck and began hauling lumber. The trucks (and their heaters) grew larger, and helped support his family for almost seventy years.

I was a bit disappointed; the story wasn't exactly dramatic stuff. But when I thought about it, I realized why Glen was fighting so hard to tell it to me. Having his own truck led to his business, his independent life, a small house in the Adirondacks, where, as he put it, he could "always put the food on the table for my family." It was one of the most important stories of his life, and of his death.

The day after Glen's memorial, Ann e-mailed me a message. I keep it taped on the wall above my computer:

"Izzy helps my heart heal. I have so many beautiful memories of you, Izzy, and myself. The most beautiful being the day Glen died. I will hold these in my heart forever. You, too, have a beautiful spirit. May God bless you abundantly. Love, Peace, and Joy to Izzy and you, as you continue with God's work."

I read and reread the message; I cherished

it. There was no pretense in that small living room, no hiding or posturing. I was as naked and exposed as Glen was, our souls revealed, stripped finally of all the pain and guile and confusion of life.

And what was left was good. It helped to hear that. I felt as if an unseen presence within me had finally shown itself and come out to live in the world.

It was a message I'd been seeking most of my life, but was always afraid to believe. This time I did believe it, and I would cling to it until it was my turn to be on the other side of the bedrails. When I get there, I hope there will be a dog to help heal my heart. And a good man or woman to bring him.

At the memorial, Ann had spoken about Glen, his gentle spirit and upright life. She said she was grateful to hospice, and to Izzy and to me. "They came into our lives when we needed them. I don't know what we would have done without them," she told the small gathering. "They lifted us like a cloud." And for the first time in all that long, confusing year, I cried.

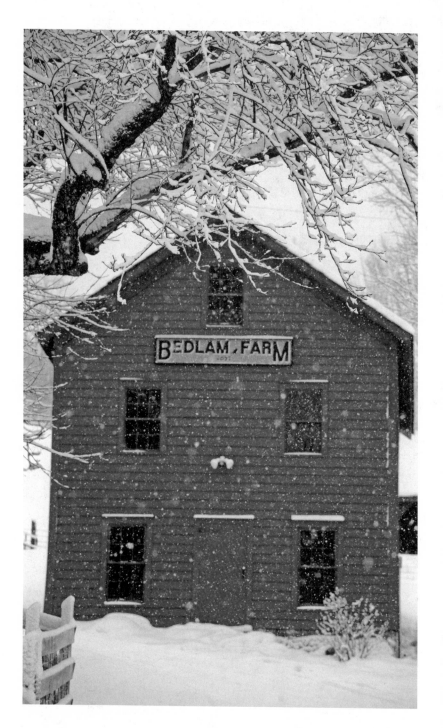

CHAPTER SIXTEEN:
FIASCO AND BLISS

What Joseph Campbell never tells you is whether mythic heroes get depressed. Do they stay awake night after night, sleeplessly fretting about their mental states or their blood sugar or the settings on their digital cameras? Or singing softly to Lab puppies?

But, like Campbell, I've come to believe that a good and worthy life consists of one hero's excursion after another.

Over and over again, Campbell wrote in his book *Pathways to Bliss: Mythology and Personal Transformation,* we are called to the realm of adventure, exploration, and rebirth; we are called to new horizons. Each time, he says, there is the same question: "Do I dare?"

If you do dare, Campbell says, there is always the possibility of fiasco.

But there is always, also, the possibility of bliss.

I did dare. I had experienced fiasco; I was

approaching, rather slowly, bliss.

I'd returned to therapy, after many years, to finally take on the demons and memories that had haunted and plagued me for so long. It is never too late, I told myself, to get better. And I was getting better, every day. All that struggle was paying off.

I was tough, after all, and wily. I understood that my greatest weapons were determination and faith.

I kept faith, even when people I loved lost it, even though I didn't deserve it, even though I couldn't understand it. Perhaps that's the true power of faith — you hold on to it when you don't know why or how it's there.

I chose to believe that I would come through, more or less intact, if not entirely whole. I threw everything I had into the fray — books, an iPod, my camera, all my energy and strength. When I wasn't reading, I was riding around the countryside, taking pictures with Izzy. When I wasn't taking pictures, I was calling my friends and family — now, once more, including my sister — to talk things over. When I wasn't doing those things, I was visiting hospice patients. Or — my latest adventure — teaching writing in a public high school. I even wrote a poem or two.

It seems to be working, and I am humbled and chastened, yet strangely proud of myself.

Taking photos like mad, posting them on my website, I got an e-mail message from a well-known photographer who told me that what matters isn't what the camera sees, but what you see. That winter, I realized he was telling the truth — there is beauty in small and common things.

Here is the fiasco: Damage was done to me, and I did damage to others. The voices in my head remind me that some conflicts are never completely won; they shift to new battlefields. I am weary. And I am sorry. I've come to see myself as battling mental illness, and it's a tough fight, with some casualties. I've experienced pain and sadness, humiliation and loss.

Here is the bliss: My creative self has helped me heal and grow stronger, and shown me that I can write a poem, take a decent photograph, tell people what I'm going through and see them turn not away but toward me.

I think of Churchill often — I even named a rooster after him. Sometimes I picture him coming to visit the farm on a summer evening; we sit on the front porch, sharing cigars and snifters of brandy and war stories.

Sacrifice and more sacrifice. Pain and more pain. The only way through hell is hell.

I love all those hoary old clichés, because so many of them are true.

The days have begun lengthening again. Late one February afternoon I made my farm rounds: cookies for the donkey, an apple for Elvis, a scattering of corn for Winston and his tribe.

The light was fading by then. Soon I'd prepare dinner for myself and for the dogs, stoke the woodstove, and we'd all settle in for the night. I'd give each dog a frozen marrow bone, and they'd find nooks and nests to retreat to with their prizes. I loved the sound of all that crunching and slurping in the corners of the old farmhouse as I read. In a while, all of us tired, we'd be dozing by the stove, at peace.

Being at peace is okay, a good thing. It had been a long time since I'd felt it, and I craved it. I was excited about things: pictures I wanted to take, classes I wanted to teach, books I wanted to write, things I wanted to do with Paula. But I was also looking forward to being able to do not much at all, to meet up with tranquillity once more. Perhaps tonight by the firelight.

First, though, the dogs needed their last

walk of the day. Izzy and Rose and Lenore and I took the trail down through the woods. As we moved deeper into the forest and the moon rose, I had a sense of something lifting and I remembered that this was what hope felt like.

My heart shifted a bit, and I knew that I would one day have my life back, or a better version of it, if I were patient and humble, worked hard and kept faith.

Lenore and Izzy bounded ahead, investigating some strange sound. But Rose waited, unusually, staring at me with her intense, beautiful eyes.

"It's okay," I told her. "It's okay." She held my gaze for a moment, then dashed off down the path to be with the other dogs.

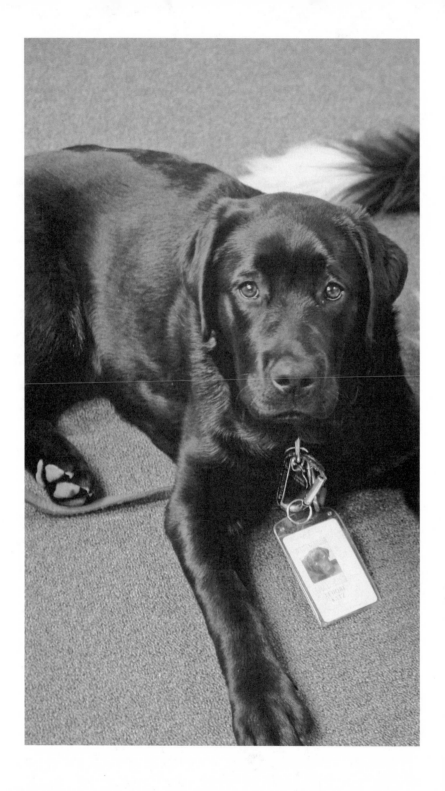

AFTERWORD

Of all the remarkable things that have happened since I moved to Bedlam Farm, none had a more powerful or lasting impact than the hospice work I did with Izzy. Nothing I saw was more mysterious or moving than the emotions dogs can evoke, their capacity to help heal us.

All winter, Izzy and I went in and out of houses and trailers and nursing homes, visiting people who were dying, and their families. And a practice that began as an impulse to do something good with my dog evolved into something much more, an excursion into the enigmatic realm of dogs and healing.

All kinds of people — rich and poor, educated and not, clearheaded and mired in pain — believed that Izzy could, not cure them, but make them feel more peaceful, loved, cared for.

What, I often wondered, is the healing

power of dogs? How does Izzy do what he does? Was it a gift, an instinct, some projection of human values onto an animal? A myth?

I read many of the slew of books, articles, and studies about dogs as aids to human health, and found little in the way of consensus or understanding. Great numbers of people believe animals have restorative abilities; it's a cherished belief. The notion of the healing animal, the animal with the mystical or spiritual power to help humankind, is ancient; it abounds in myths, cave drawings, stories, and legends. Many of us still want to believe in it.

The scientific and behavioral evidence is fuzzy, though. A number of studies show that people with animals live a bit longer and are somewhat healthier — they get more exercise, and have marginally better blood pressure and heart rates than people who don't live with animals. But that's about as far as the consensus goes.

And that's okay by me. Frankly, I like the mystery of it. The dog world already has too many experts and gurus. Some aspects of dogs and other animals simply lie beyond the comprehension of humans, who aren't blessed with nearly as many useful instincts.

It seems clear that animals' presence in

nursing homes, hospitals, and schools, where they can work with adults and children with a wide variety of illnesses, disabilities, and emotional problems, can have real emotional impact. They soothe people, make them feel better, make them smile.

Some scientists believe that dogs, with their keen senses, can smell sickness and pain, and in some fashion intuit need. Perhaps they connect in some spiritual way we can't see or understand.

Our era has seen the advent of the therapy dog, who interacts with sick or damaged people. Nobody knows how many therapy dogs are on the job, but they're increasingly prevalent.

More broadly, we believe dogs can help us in lots of ways. We think they can see and hear and sense things that are beyond us. We believe they can find us when we're lost, track down evildoers, protect us from hidden bombs, as well as serve as our emotional companions and supports. The idea of the healing dog is an attractive one in our busy, fragmented society.

Still, I was surprised again and again by Izzy and the work he did. I remember his impact on Etta, the elderly nursing-home resident suffering from cancer and dementia, who barely seemed to notice Izzy, who at first swatted him away. When she felt his head beneath her hand, she calmed visibly.

I think of Paul, another dementia patient, who actually began to speak after a few Izzy visits, and left the hospice rolls. And, of course, I recall Glen, the logging trucker, for whom Izzy was a pathway to his own life and grief, and a helpful companion at the end of his life.

I wasn't sure, when we began, how Izzy would interact with the dying, or how they would respond to him. I'd trained him to be calm, obedient, and focused on me, but there was no way I could have trained him to be sensitive to the needs of people in pain, on medication, tethered to equipment, facing their deaths.

Anxious about what we might encounter, I was prepared to pull out at any time, drop the idea, leave the dog at home.

But Izzy seemed to grasp what was needed. We would enter a house, and he would scan the room, watching me closely for some cue. Early on, he was drawn to the first person who reacted to him or spoke to him — it might be the hospice nurse, a family member, or a friend. He seemed a bit puzzled as to why he was there, and looked to me for direction.

It was some time before I grasped the extent to which this was work for him, work we were doing together, in almost the same way Rose and I herded sheep. Izzy was the one connecting with the patients; but he could accomplish this because of our relationship. I was not, as I often joked, just Izzy's driver.

I began to give him unspoken signals, almost unconsciously at first, later with some thought and care. I went over to the patient, touched him or her, and encouraged Izzy to come over. When he did, I praised him, reinforcing the behavior, telling him he was a good dog, telling him to stay.

Izzy is a calm guy but he pays rapt attention. Once he had cues, he followed them. When they paid off, he incorporated them into his work.

I've had many gentle, well-trained dogs, but none who could be as delicate and intuitive. I believe he observed me for instructions, read my responses, and began to respond to reinforcement from me, from the patients, from their families. I was impressed, and a bit relieved.

Izzy developed a sense for who the patient was. I think he came to look for a bed or wheelchair, or for a person lying down. Over time, perhaps, he also learned to recognize the medical detritus that surrounds patients — the pills, oxygen tanks, hospital beds.

He also, I'm sure, sensed something in the bearing, the movements, or the smells of the dying, things humans can't always detect. Often their voices were distinct, weaker, softer; perhaps he noticed. They responded differently to Izzy than other people did, too; they were more focused on him, more aware of him, and their exclamations of joy, pleasure, even relief, at seeing him must have sounded unlike other people's.

We often underestimate the strength of the signals that pass between dog and human, and I sometimes underrate the extent to which my dogs read my moods and feelings. Yet it's there, evident when I'm sheepherding with Rose, tossing a ball for Lenore, and especially when I'm taking Izzy to a hospice home.

How could he fail to pick up on my awe for his instincts, my love and appreciation for what he was doing? And the other people in the room — the patient and family members, the hospice staff — felt the same way. So Izzy, a sensitive sort, was dramatically, repeatedly reinforced for his behavior, and quickly figured out what was expected.

And yet, this was no mere training exercise, with commands and rewards. What was going on inside him was less clear. After our hospice visits, I noticed Izzy seemed spent;

sometimes he hardly moved for the rest of the day. It was tiring work for him, I could see, even if it wasn't physical. It took a lot of canine energy, in ways I couldn't fathom.

Undeniably, the work caused us to bond in an extraordinary way. My relationship with Izzy grew deeper and richer, and it was sometimes difficult to disentangle my own feelings from his instincts. This was a remarkable experience for a human and a dog, satisfying beyond words. I wish I could better describe the almost physical sensation of admiration that came from watching this dog do his work.

I have no doubt that Izzy was healing me as well as helping the dying. Each visit settled me, grounded me, rewarded me. Izzy surely would have picked up on that as well. He has a great heart; he lives to serve people.

He taught me, too. By even the second or third hospice visit, I felt clearer about my task, more confident. I, too, now walked right up to the patient, touched him, spoke to him, sat by the bed or chair, focused my attention. Both of us volunteers improved in our ability to help.

Often Izzy and I would split up: He took care of the patient, I turned to the spouse or family member, often a person struggling mightily with fear, exhaustion, and impending grief. We made a difference, we knew it, could feel it, and we left those homes with a sense of perspective, accomplishment, well-being. What could be more healing than that?

I often wondered, though, why a dog's presence meant so much to people at the end of their lives. Presumably, they had many other things to think about — their pasts, the friends and family they were leaving behind, what lay ahead.

It was perhaps the murkiest part of the experience for me. So often I saw that time with Izzy mattered to people who were dying, even if they weren't fully conscious or aware.

Part of it, I could see, was a need for love without reservations. Izzy simply loved them and accepted them, no matter what they looked like, smelled like, felt like. They didn't have to talk to Izzy, impress him, explain themselves, exert themselves. They could simply touch and hold him.

I think Izzy served as an emotional channel as well. I don't know how or why, but I saw it: Izzy allowed access to feelings people wouldn't or couldn't express to other people. The dog opened a door, and all sorts of things poured through it — grief, fear, memories, laughter.

Sometimes spouses and children couldn't bear to face or discuss death; sometimes the dying didn't want to burden their loved ones with their feelings. Sometimes they were afraid to talk openly to doctors or nurses or volunteers, because they didn't want to cause trouble, be a bother, or get sent to a nursing home or hospital.

Izzy, however, was happy to be with dying people, to hear whatever they wanted to say. Their grief and their sadness or regret, their quiet but urgent efforts to come to terms with their deaths — he never turned away from any of it.

Over time, I came to believe that his silent companionship allowed people to be contemplative and exploratory. The process that social workers called "venting" — ventilating feelings — was enabled and accelerated by a creature so nonjudgmental, so easy to talk to. I couldn't say exactly how this worked, but I saw it happen.

Through hospice, I recognized how fearful death is in our culture — so repressed that people flee from seeing it, thinking about it, accepting it.

Izzy had no such cultural bias. The dying were merely people who welcomed him, and all sorts of emotions emerged as they became comfortable with him, ruffled his soft fur, felt his warmth and affection. He was not afraid of death, and I think the people he saw especially appreciated that.

Izzy couldn't communicate in human terms, but his bearing and demeanor spoke for him. He was saying: I'm just here visiting, providing some comfort. I don't ask anything, except to be here next to you.

At times something so palpable passed between Izzy and these people that it awed, even disturbed, me, because I couldn't understand it or explain it. These were humbling moments, spiritual, beyond my experience or comprehension. Several times I felt I was in the presence of something much mightier than the two of us, that I was meant to be in that room, to witness those events for a reason.

The reason seemed to be that I was there to help, to comfort, and to be helped and comforted. And Izzy was the vessel, the vehicle, the spirit that could guide us there.

I seek to be a spiritual man, but I'm not deeply or conventionally religious. I was born a Jew; I became a Quaker; I wear the cross. I don't know, really, what I am, in terms of labels.

But going into those houses, seeing people moving swiftly toward the end of their lives, I had no trouble feeling and believing in a meaning greater than Izzy or me, or any of us.

After the people we visited had died, their families invariably asked me to bring Izzy back to say good-bye. So an additional ritual developed: Izzy walked into the home, or the room, accepted everyone's pats and hugs, then moved to the very spot where he'd last seen the patient. He hopped up onto the bed or sofa and lay there, quite still, for perhaps ten or fifteen minutes. He closed his eyes and went to sleep, paying scant attention to me, the family, or anyone else in the room.

I sat and talked a while, usually, and when I was ready to leave, Izzy jumped down and walked out the door. He didn't look back. In all honesty, I can't guess what this was about. It looked as if he was saying good-bye, going to the last places he had seen his friends, communicating with them in some unknowable way. Maybe he expected them to return, or was seeking a scent, a presence.

I don't know. I will never know, and I don't believe anyone knows. For all of the expertise in this world, some things are beyond our studies and reports, beyond our ability to know or grasp. You just have to leave it there. At least I do.

Izzy is an intuitive creature. He sees things I don't see, hears things I don't hear, feels things I'll never feel. He comforts, if not heals; he calms, if not cures. He's a doorway to humans' deepest feelings and emotions at perhaps the most critical point in their lives.

I love the mystery of him. Sometimes, after our visits, I pulled the car over and took his head in my hands, looked into his eyes, hugged him tightly. He always leaned against me, returning my love but revealing and explaining nothing — nothing but affection, connection, faithfulness.

I could take him to a thousand homes, I realize, and never really grasp just what he's doing or why, or the reasons people find it meaningful. They just do, and that's enough.

I believe Izzy may be a spirit dog, one of those guides that the ancients drew pictures of on cave walls. He inhabits another realm. He came to me, in that circuitous way, for a purpose, and the purpose is revealed in houses and trailers and nursing homes.

Late one winter afternoon, sitting in the darkness, I watched Izzy lying next to Timmy in his hospital bed. This dying little boy, his mother, the house — the world was still in that moment. I saw Izzy open his eyes, raise his head, and look at me sitting in a chair halfway across the room.

I didn't want to awaken the mother, who was dozing nearby on the sofa, or disturb the boy, who looked peaceful, his arm draped over Izzy's shoulder. In so awful and unnatural a scene, there could still be a quiet, restful moment.

Izzy has no supernatural powers. He could not heal that boy, or ease his pain, or alter the course of his life, any more than doctors and medicines could. Timmy would die shortly, and we weren't there to stop that. There was no stopping it.

Still, this was a scene I wouldn't forget, and which I felt awed to witness.

I looked Izzy in the eye and thought, but didn't speak, these words: Be still, boy, don't move. He needs you to lie right where you are for a while, so both these weary people can have some rest. That's why we're here.

Izzy met my gaze and held it for a bit, then laid his head back down on Timmy's shoulder.

I doubt many things. I am absolutely sure of nothing, especially at the end of this year. But I know for sure that my dog — who had known abandonment, hunger, loneliness, and pain himself — heard every word I didn't say.

POSTSCRIPT

I was wrong about Lenore.

A few months after I decided she wasn't destined for hospice work, I went to visit a friend whose mother was quite ill. She was a dog lover, my friend said, so I brought Lenore, a proven spirits-booster.

I watched her sidle up to the woman and gently offer her love and attention, and began to wonder. Perhaps what I'd seen before was just boisterous puppyhood. Perhaps Lenore, so affectionate by nature, might yet have potential.

I began intensive calming training; we practiced sit-downs and stays, lie-downs and get-backs. Meanwhile, I continued taking Lenore to stores, doctors' offices, and hospice meetings.

In February, she sailed through a rigorous temperament test with flying colors. On March 1, she undertook her first hospice assignment, visiting an elderly man with congestive heart failure.

Lenore was extraordinary: calm, appropriate, responsive. She did the job, brightening the room with her sweet nature and great heart. What a thrill to see the working dog emerge in this profoundly loving creature.

It remains to be seen whether Lenore has Izzy's intuitive touch, or whether she'll bring a different kind of comfort. Either way, our hospice team has doubled, and I'm proud of her.

PASSAGE
Mary Kellogg

I look into the eyes
of
vagueness
but still life and warmth of body
focusing on what we can not see

seeing beyond the blue vase with flowers
the open bible on the shelf
the bent head
cheeks wet with tears

we wait for the moment
this time is now

no more than a sigh
a step over into calm

where does it begin and where does it end
that moment when night becomes dawn
when the tide turns

and finds you

a heart open to love
cradling the passage

January 2008
North Hebron, New York

For more information about hospice care, or to locate a hospice organization near you, contact the National Hospice and Palliative Care Organization at www.nhpco.org. It operates a helpline at 800-568-8898.

ABOUT THE AUTHOR

Jon Katz has written seventeen books — six novels and eleven works of nonfiction — including *Dog Days, A Dog Year, The New Work of Dogs, The Dogs of Bedlam Farm,* and *Katz on Dogs.* A two-time finalist for the National Magazine Award, he has written for *The New York Times, The Wall Street Journal, Rolling Stone,* and the *AKC Gazette.* A member of the Association of Pet Dog Trainers, he writes columns about dogs and rural life for the online magazine *Slate* and cohosts the award-winning radio show *Dog Talk* on Northeast Public Radio. Also a photographer, Katz lives on Bedlam Farm in upstate New York with his wife, Paula Span, and his dogs, sheep, goats, donkeys, barn cats, irritable rooster Winston, and three hens. Visit hospice@bedlamfarm.com, www.bedlamfarm.com, and www.photosby jonkatz.com.